D0897728 ACL9W

EUROPEAN
SOCIETY OF
CARDIOLOGY

The evaluation
and treatment
of syncope

A handbook for clinical practice

The evaluation and treatment of syncope

A handbook for clinical practice

A publication based on the
Guidelines on Management (diagnosis and treatment) of Syncope
by the European Society of Cardiology (see our website at
http://www.escardio.org/scinfo/Tforceguidelines.htm#Syncope)

EDITED BY

David G Benditt MD, FACC, FRCP(C)

Jean-Jacques Blanc MD, FESC

Michele Brignole MD, FESC

Richard Sutton DSc Med, FRCP, FESC, FACC

FUTURA

Blackwell
Publishing

Futura, an imprint of Blackwell Publishing

© 2003 European Society of Cardiology
2035 Route des Colles-Les Templiers, 06903 Sophia-Antipolis, France
For further information on the European Society of Cardiology,
visit our website: www.escardio.org

Published by Futura, an imprint of Blackwell Publishing
Blackwell Publishing, Inc./Futura Division, 3 West Main Street, Elmsford,
   New York 10523, USA
Blackwell Publishing, Inc., 350 Main Street, Malden, Massachusetts 02148-5020,
   USA
Blackwell Publishing Ltd, 9600 Garsington Road, Oxford OX4 2DQ
Blackwell Science Asia Pty Ltd, 550 Swanston Street, Carlton, Victoria 3053,
   Australia

03 04 05 06 5 4 3 2 1

ISBN: 1-4051-0374-4

Catalogue records for this title are available from the British Library and Library of
Congress

Acquisitions: Jacques Strauss
Production: Julie Elliott
Typesetter: Graphicraft Ltd., Hong Kong
Printed and bound by MPG Books Ltd, Bodmin, Cornwall, UK

For further information on Blackwell Publishing, visit our website:
www.futuraco.com
www.blackwellpublishing.com

Contents

Section three: Guide to selection of diagnostic procedures

Section four: Causes of syncope and syncope mimics, and treatment

List of contributors

*Member of the ESC Management of Syncope Task Force

Editors

David G Benditt, MD, FACC, FRCP(C), Cardiac Arrhythmia Center, Department of Medicine, Cardiovascular Division, University of Minnesota, Minneapolis, USA*
Jean-Jacques Blanc, MD, FESC, Département de Cardiologie, Hôpital de la Cavale Blanche, CHU de Brest, France*
Michele Brignole, MD, FESC, Department of Cardiology and Arrhythmologic Centre, Ospedali del Tigullio, Lavagna, Italy*
Richard Sutton, DSc Med, FRCP, FESC, FACC, Department of Cardiology, Royal Brompton Hospital, London, UK*

Contributors

Paolo Alboni, MD, FACC, Divisione di Cardiologia, Ospedale Civile, Cento, Italy*
Lennart Bergfeldt, MD, PhD, FESC, Electrophysiology & Arrhythmia Service, Department of Cardiology, Thoracic Clinics, Karolinska Hospital Stockholm, Sweden*
J Gert van Dijk, MD, PhD, Department of Neurology and Clinical Neurophysiology, Leiden University Medical Centre, Leiden, The Netherlands *
Adam P Fitzpatrick, MD, FRCP, FACC, Manchester Heart Centre, Manchester Royal Infirmary, Manchester, UK and Manor Lodge Consulting Centre, Cheadle, UK*
Karin S Ganzeboom, BS, Department of Medicine, Academic Medical Centre, University of Amsterdam, Amsterdam, The Netherlands
Jan Janousek, MD, Kardiocentrum, University Hospital Motol, Prague, Czech Republic*
Wishwa N Kapoor, MD, MPH, Department of Internal Medicine, University of Pittsburgh, Pittsburgh, Pennsylvania, USA*
Rose Anne Kenny, MD, FESC, Institute for the Health of the Elderly, University of Newcastle Upon Tyne, Royal,Victoria Infirmary, Newcastle upon Tyne, UK*
Piotr Kulakowski, MD, FESC, Department of Cardiology, Medical Centre of Postgraduate Education, Grochowski Hospital, Warsaw, Poland*
Johannes J van Lieshout, MD, PhD, Department of Medicine, Academic Medical Centre, University of Amsterdam, Amsterdam, The Netherlands
Fei Lu, MD, PhD, Cardiac Arrhythmia Center, Department of Medicine, Cardiovascular Division, University of Minnesota, Minneapolis, USA
Angel Moya, MD, FESC, Department of Cardiology, Hospital General Vall d'Hebron, Barcelona, Spain*
Antonio Raviele, MD, FESC, Divisione di Cardiologia, Ospedale Umberto I, Mestre-Venice, Italy*
Robert Sheldon, MD, PhD, FRCP(C), Cardiovascular Research Group, Division of Cardiology, University of Calgary, Calgary, Alberta, Canada
George Theodorakis, MD, FESC, 2° Department of Cardiology, Onassis Cardiac Surgery Center, Athens, Greece*
Wouter Wieling, MD, PhD, Department of Medicine, Academic Medical Centre, University of Amsterdam, Amsterdam, The Netherlands*

Contributors
European Heart House,
Nice, France, 2002

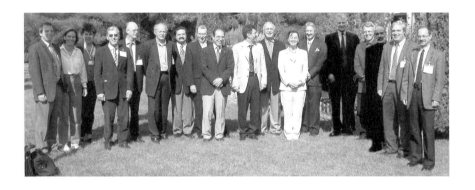

From left to right

Robert Sheldon, MD, PhD, FRCP(C)
Veronica Dean (ESC Staff)
Dominique Poumeyrol-Jumeau (ESC Staff)
Paolo Alboni, MD, FACC
J Gert van Dijk, MD, PhD
Wouter Wieling, MD, PhD
Angel Moya, MD, FESC
Jean-Jacques Blanc, MD, FESC
Antonio Raviele, MD, FESC
Michele Brignole, MD, FESC
David G Benditt, MD, FACC, FRCP(C)
Rose Anne Kenny, MD, FESC

Richard Sutton, DSc Med, FRCP, FESC, FACC
Adam P Fitzpatrick, MD, FRCP, FACC
Lennart Bergfeldt, MD, PhD, FESC
Wishwa N Kapoor, MD MPH
George Theodorakis, MD, FESC
Piotr Kulakowski, MD, FESC

Not shown
Jan Janousek, MD
Karin S Ganzeboom, BS
Johannes J van Lieshout, MD, PhD
Fei Lu, MD, PhD

Introduction

Michele Brignole

This handbook is based on the published *Guidelines on the Management (Diagnosis and Treatment) of Syncope* of the European Society of Cardiology. The contributors are primarily comprised of Task Force members. The purpose was principally to provide a means for disseminating the *Guidelines* in a manner that was readily accessible to medical professionals, and could be conveniently utilized in the office, clinic and emergency department.

The Task Force was constituted in 1999 and the first edition of the *Guidelines* was published in 2001 (*Eur Heart J* 2001; 22: 1256–1306). The purpose of these guidelines is to provide specific recommendations on the diagnostic evaluation and management of syncope. The creation of a panel of experts was justified by the fact that in this field data from the literature are often not definitive, and a lack of standardization exists regarding the appropriate strategy for diagnostic procedures and their interpretation. There are several reasons for this. First, a major issue in the use of diagnostic tests is that syncope is a transient symptom and not a disease. Typically patients are most often asymptomatic at the time of evaluation. The opportunity to capture a spontaneous event during diagnostic testing is rare. As a result, the diagnostic evaluation must focus on discerning susceptibility to physiologic states that could cause loss of consciousness. This type of reasoning leads, of necessity, to uncertainty in establishing a cause. In other words, the causal relationship between a diagnostic abnormality and syncope in a given patient is often presumptive. Second, in the absence of documentation at the time of an event, the establishment of the cause of syncope depends critically on taking an accurate and detailed history. Currently, there is a great deal of variation in how physicians take the history and their knowledge base regarding the crucial information for which to seek and its interpretation. Third, since documentation of spontaneous syncope events is relatively rare, measurements of test sensitivity are not possible. Essentially, there is lack of a gold standard for most of the tests employed for this condition. Most of the time decisions have to be made based on a patient's history or abnormal findings during asymptomatic periods. To overcome the lack of a gold standard, the diagnostic yield of many tests in syncope has been assessed indirectly by the evaluation of the reduction of syncopal recurrences after administration of the specific therapy suggested by the results of the test which were "diagnostic." In the absence of randomized controlled treatment trials, inferences derived from follow-up observations is inherently suspect.

Given these issues the objectives of the Task Force were to provide:
- criteria for diagnosis of the cause of syncope from history and physical examination;
- guidelines for choosing tests and determining test abnormalities in the further evaluation of syncope;
- advice regarding how to use the results of diagnostic procedures in defining the most probable cause of syncope; and
- recommendations regarding the most appropriate treatment strategy.

The methodology for writing the basic Guideline document consisted of literature reviews and consensus development by the panel. The recommendations provided in this book are directly derived from that development process. However, since the goal of the book was to provide practicable specific recommendations for diagnosis and management for practicing care-givers, recommendations are often provided even when the data from the literature are not definitive. In fact, as remains the case in much of medical practice, most of the recommendations are based on consensus expert opinion.

In order to facilitate reading, this handbook provides neither levels of evidence for every recommendation, nor literature citations for each statement. Key goals for each section are noted at the beginning of that section. Additional reading for each section will be found at the end of each segment of the text. Further, a relatively complete literature source, divided into major interest areas (e.g., pathophysiology, history-taking, tilt-table testing) is provided separately at the end of the volume. The interested reader is referred to the *European Society of Cardiology Guidelines* document for statements of levels of evidence and detailed literature citations (you can download this document from the guidelines section of our website: www.escardio.org/scinfo/guidelines.htm).

The reader will find in this handbook practical consideration of the most important clinical aspects related to the evaluation and treatment of patients with syncope:
- What are the diagnostic criteria for causes of syncope?
- What is the preferred approach to the diagnostic work-up in various subgroups of patients with syncope?
- How should patients with syncope be risk stratified?
- When should patients with syncope be hospitalized?
- Which treatments are likely to be effective in preventing syncope recurrences?

This book attempts to present this information in a succinct form. It is directed toward practicing physicians who encounter syncope patients. Thus, we envision it being widely useful. It should have particular value to practitioners in emergency medicine, primary care, internal medicine, neurology, pediatrics and cardiology.

The Guidelines document and this handbook owe their development to many individuals who planned the tasks, undertook the research, wrote the text, and provided the financial resources to bring these efforts to fruition. The authors particularly appreciate the encouragement and support provided by the leadership and staff of the European Society of Cardiology, and specifically the chairman of the Committee for Practice Guidelines, Professor Werner Klein (2000–2002), his coordinating secretary, Ms Veronica Dean and her assistant Ms Dominique Poumeyrol-Jumeau.

We are also grateful to St Jude Medical Inc. (St Paul, MN) for a grant in support of this publication, and to Medtronic Inc. (Minneapolis, MN) for a grant in support of the consensus conference at which many of the recommendations in this publication were solidified.

Section one:
Definition, pathophysiology, epidemiology

CHAPTER 1

Syncope: definition, classification, and multiple potential causes

Jean-Jacques Blanc, David G Benditt

Introduction

The term "syncope" is derived from an old Greek word meaning "to cut short" or "interrupt". In modern usage, it refers to interruption of global cerebral activity resulting in loss of consciousness. In this case, however, it implies a transient reversible condition. Thus syncope refers to a symptomatic episode in which loss of consciousness occurs, but is temporary and self-terminating. However, English-speaking patients rarely use the word "syncope". More commonly they will talk of "fainting" or "blacking out", "passing out" or, in former days, "swooning". Syncope must be considered as part of the differential diagnosis for patients who present with an apparent self-limited "fall" or "collapse" (Fig. 1.1).

The principal mechanism underlying any type of faint is a transient diminution of blood flow to the brain, such that a disturbance of global cerebral

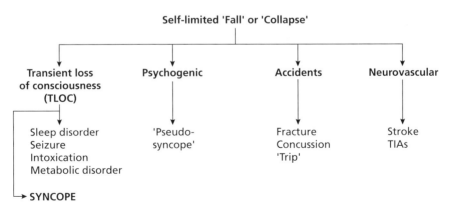

Fig. 1.1 Scheme depicting differential diagnostic considerations for patients who present with a self-limited fall or collapse. Syncope is only one element of the differential, but is the primary focus of this book.

Table 1.1 Other conditions often
mistakenly considered to be syncope.

Dizziness
Vertigo
Drop attacks
Falls
Psychogenic syncope
Transient ischemic attack (TIA)

function occurs (see Chapter 2). As discussed below, this definition eliminates many other conditions that are often mistakenly considered to be syncope (Table 1.1).

Goals

This chapter provides an introduction to the concept of syncope as a symptom (not a diagnosis) with multiple potential causes. Indeed, multiple possibilities frequently coexist in the same patient, thereby complicating the diagnostic dilemma. Specifically, the objectives of this section are to:
• define syncope;
• provide a classification of the principal causes of syncope in a manner that we hope will be clinically useful; and
• highlight the possibility that multiple potential contributing factors need to be considered when evaluating syncope patients.

Definition

Syncope is a symptom defined as a transient, self-limited loss of consciousness, and as a consequence the concomitant loss of voluntary muscle tone. The onset of syncope is relatively rapid and the subsequent recovery is spontaneous, complete and usually prompt. The underlying mechanism is transient global cerebral hypoperfusion.

Elements of the definition of syncope
The definition of syncope incorporates five main components. Each of these must be fulfillled before one can establish that "true" syncope has occurred.

Loss of consciousness
This is a major element which has to be discovered by the history taken from the patient or from those who witnessed the episode. If there is no loss of consciousness, the diagnosis of syncope is excluded—it is something else. Table 1.1 gives some examples of the most common misdiagnoses.

Consider for example transient ischemic attacks (TIAs). For many physicians, TIAs are thought to be a common cause of syncope but, in fact, syncope is in practical terms never the consequence of TIA. This is a crucial issue as many commonly ordered diagnostic tests (e.g., head CT or MRI scan, carotid Doppler evaluation) are prescribed on the basis of looking for the origin of a presumed TIA. In fact, these are almost always a waste of resources. To summarize, during a TIA the patient loses something: motility, vision, speech—but never consciousness. In other words, syncope is transient loss of consciousness without localizing neurologic deficit, while a TIA is transient loss of focal neurologic function without loss of consciousness.

Loss of voluntary muscle tone
Loss of voluntary muscle control is inherent to loss of consciousness. Therefore, if standing, the fainter falls down; if seated he or she slumps over.

Onset is relatively rapid
By definition, a faint is a temporary loss of consciousness. As a rule the onset is rapid, being no more than 10–20 sec after onset of premonitory symptoms (if there are any such symptoms). Faints may be associated with any of a variety of warning symptoms (or none at all), and the nature of these, as determined by the initial evaluation and medical history-taking (Chapter 5), may provide important clues as to the cause of the symptoms. On the other hand, many fainters either do not experience or are unaware of any premonitory symptoms. This lack of warning seems to be particularly prevalent in older individuals. Among patients who do experience warning symptoms, symptoms are often reported as a feeling of "lightheadedness" or a "dizziness" as the faint evolves. Additionally they may experience progressive darkening or "graying-out" of vision, and progressive hearing impairment. Depending on the specific situation, other warning symptoms may include a sense of rapid or irregular heart rhythm, nausea, sweating and variable "hot–cold" sensation.

Recovery is spontaneous, complete and usually prompt
This aspect of the definition excludes a number of conditions which result in loss of consciousness, but which in fact do not reverse themselves to normal in the absence of medical intervention. Examples of such conditions are coma (particularly hypoglycemia), intoxicated states (alcohol, narcotics, other drugs) and stroke.

Underlying mechanism is transient global cerebral hypoperfusion
This element of pathophysiology differentiates "true syncope" from seizures (epilepsy). The latter does lead to loss of consciousness with complete and spontaneous recovery, but its origin is not inadequacy of cerebral perfusion.

Table 1.2 summarizes the main differences between syncope and epilepsy. Perhaps the aspect of greatest importance in this regard is abnormal motor activity. In syncope, it is not uncommon for patients to exhibit jerky movements of the arms and legs for a brief period of time. These movements may

Table 1.2 Distinguishing syncope from seizures.

Clinical findings that suggest the diagnosis	Seizure likely	Syncope likely
Symptoms before the event	Blue face Aura (such as funny smell)	Nausea, vomiting, abdominal discomfort, feeling of cold, sweating (neurally mediated)
Findings during loss of consciousness (as observed by an eye-witness)	Tonic–clonic movements are usually prolonged and their onset coincides with loss of consciousness (< 15 sec) Hemilateral clonic movement Clear automatisms such as chewing or lip smacking or frothing at the mouth Tongue biting	Jerky movements are always of short duration and they start after the loss of consciousness
Symptoms after the event	Prolonged confusion Aching muscles *Other clinical findings of less value for suspecting seizure (low specificity)* Family history Timing of the event (night) Lightheadedness before the event "Pins and needles" before the event Incontinence after the event Injury after the event Headache after the event Sleepiness after the event	Usually short duration Nausea, vomiting, pallor (neurally mediated)

be interpreted by nonexpert bystanders as a "seizure" or a "fit". However, the jerky movements during a faint differ from those accompanying a grand mal epileptic seizure in several ways. They are briefer, they tend to occur after the loss of consciousness has set in, and they are more jerky and do not have the "tonic–clonic" features of a true grand mal epileptic seizure. Similarly, loss of bowel control commonly seen with seizures is rare during a faint. Bladder control may be lost in both cases, but is less common in fainters.

Causes of syncope: classification and single versus multiple etiologies

Table 1.3 provides a classification of the causes of syncope beginning with the most frequently encountered conditions, the neurally mediated reflex faints. However, it should be borne in mind that even after a thorough assessment, it

Table 1.3 Syncope classification.

Neurally mediated reflex syncopal syndromes
Vasovagal faint (common faint)
Carotid sinus syncope
Situational faint
  Acute hemorrhage
  Cough, sneeze
  Gastrointestinal stimulation (swallow, defecation, visceral pain)
  Micturition (postmicturition)
  Postexercise
  Other (e.g., brass instrument playing, weightlifting, postprandial)
Glossopharyngeal and trigeminal neuralgia

Orthostatic
Primary autonomic failure syndromes (e.g., pure autonomic failure, multiple system atrophy, Parkinson's disease with autonomic failure)
Secondary autonomic failure syndromes (e.g., diabetic neuropathy, amyloid neuropathy, drugs and alcohol)
  Volume depletion
  Hemorrhage, diarrhea, Addison's disease

Cardiac arrhythmias as primary cause
Sinus node dysfunction (including bradycardia/tachycardia syndrome)
Atrioventricular conduction system disease
Paroxysmal supraventricular and ventricular tachycardias
Inherited syndromes (e.g., long QT syndrome, Brugada syndrome)
Implanted device (pacemaker, ICD) malfunction, drug-induced proarrhythmias

Structural cardiac or cardiopulmonary disease
Cardiac valvular disease
Acute myocardial infarction/ischemia
Obstructive cardiomyopathy
Atrial myxoma
Acute aortic dissection
Pericardial disease/tamponade
Pulmonary embolus/pulmonary hypertension

Cerebrovascular
Vascular steal syndromes

---

may not be possible to assign a single cause for fainting. Often patients have multiple comorbidities and as a consequence they may have several equally probable causes of fainting. Thus, individuals with severe heart disease may faint due to transient tachyarrhythmias, high-grade atrioventricular block, or even as a consequence of overmedication. Thus, the physician must not be lured into the trap of accepting an observed abnormality as either the certain cause, or even the sole cause of fainting in a given individual.

Later chapters provide a comprehensive discussion of the most important causes of syncope and their appropriate investigation. A brief overview is provided here.

Neurally mediated reflex faints are of several different types, but the best known is the common or vasovagal faint. This is the swoon often seen in films (usually triggered in the movies by a painful or emotionally upsetting event). The vasovagal faint can occur in both healthy persons as well as those with health problems; it is not indicative of nervous system disease and should not typically initiate neurologic studies. The patient experiencing a vasovagal type of reflex faint is very likely to feel nauseated and sweaty before fainting, and often appears pale and feels clammy. After the fact, they often feel tired; this sensation may last hours or days. Other reflex faints include carotid sinus syndrome, or faints triggered by micturition or defecation. Coughing, swallowing, laughing or even forcibly blowing into a wind instrument may also trigger a reflex faint.

Orthostatic (postural) faints are also common, and most often are associated with movement from lying or sitting to a standing position. Many healthy individuals experience a minor form of this faint when they need to support themselves momentarily as they stand up. However, the most dramatic postural faints occur in older frail individuals, those who have underlying medical problems (e.g., diabetes, certain nervous system diseases), or persons who are dehydrated from hot environments or inadequate fluid intake. Certain commonly prescribed medications such as diuretics, beta-adrenergic blockers, antihypertensives, or vasodilators (e.g., nitroglycerin) predispose to postural faints.

Cardiac arrhythmias may cause faints if the heart rate is too slow or too fast. Occasionally, such faints occur in otherwise healthy people such as at the onset of a paroxysmal supraventricular tachycardia (SVT) episode. However, individuals with underlying heart disease (e.g., previous myocardial infarction, valvular heart disease) are at greater risk. In either case the faint tends to occur at the onset of the rhythm problem, before compensatory vasoconstriction has a chance to respond and support the central systemic pressure. Faints may also occur when a rapid abnormal rhythm stops suddenly, and a pause ensues before the normal heart rhythm takes over again. If this is more than 5 sec in duration, the patient can experience lightheadedness or a faint (especially if they are in an upright position at the time).

Structural cardiopulmonary diseases are relatively infrequent causes of faints. The most common cause in this category is fainting associated with an acute myocardial infarction or ischemic event. The faint in this case is primarily caused by an abnormal nervous system reaction similar to the reflex faints. In general, faints caused by structural disease of the heart or blood vessels are particularly important to recognize as they are warning of potentially life-threatening conditions.

Cerebrovascular disease is rarely the cause of a faint. Perhaps subclavian steal is the best example in this class, but it is extremely uncommon. In the absence

Table 1.4 Causes of nonsyncopal attacks commonly misdiagnosed as syncope.

Disorders with impairment or loss of consciousness
Metabolic disorders, including hypoglycemia, hypoxia, hyperventilation with hypocapnia
Epilepsy
Intoxication (drugs, alcohol)
Vertebrobasilar transient ischemic attack

Disorders resembling syncope without loss of consciousness
Cataplexy
Drop attacks
Psychogenic syncope (somatization disorders)
Transient ischemic attacks of carotid artery origin

---

of clear-cut fixed or transient localizing neurologic signs during physical examination, cerebrovascular disease as a cause of syncope is unlikely. As a rule, this category should be considered only after all other "causes" have been eliminated.

Conditions that mimic faints are included here primarily because they are commonly confused with true faints (Table 1.4). As a consequence of this confusion (often aggravated by the manner in which even well-known investigators present their findings in the literature), the process needed to arrive at the correct diagnosis is impeded. The most common conditions in this category include: seizures, sleep disturbances, accidental falls and some psychiatric conditions (e.g., anxiety attacks, severe hyperventilation and hysterical reactions). Inner ear problems causing dizziness (vertigo) are also frequently mislabeled as faints. Neurologic and metabolic disturbances (such as diabetes) are rarely the cause of true fainting.

Summary

The methods recommended to determine the most probable cause of syncope and ascertain which treatment direction is most appropriate are reviewed in subsequent chapters of this book. Here we have attempted to provide an introductory overview, so that the reader will better appreciate the value of understanding the pathophysiology and the differential diagnosis. In the end, however, it is important to bear in mind that neurally mediated reflex syncope, orthostatic syncope and cardiac arrhythmias account for approximately 60–70% of the recognized causes of syncope. Further, in 20% of patients the cause of syncope remains unknown in spite of an extensive and well-planned evaluation. In some of this latter 20% there may be multiple possible causes, and distinguishing among them in an effort to find a "sole" cause may be both impossible and incorrect.

Further reading

Brignole M, Alboni P, Benditt DG *et al*. Guidelines on management (diagnosis and treatment) of syncope. *Eur Heart J* 2001; 22: 1256–1306.

Kapoor W. Evaluation and outcome of patients with syncope. *Medicine* 1990; 69: 160–175.

Benditt DG, Goldstein MA. Fainting. *Circulation* 2002; 106: 1048–1050.

Sheldon R, Rose S, Ritchie D *et al*. Historical criteria that distinguish syncope from seizures. *J Am Coll Cardiol* 2002; 40: 142–148.

Soteriades ES, Evans JC, Larson MG *et al*. Incidence and prognosis of syncope. *N Engl J Med* 2002; 347(12): 878–885.

CHAPTER 2

Pathophysiology and clinical presentation

Wouter Wieling, J Gert van Dijk, Johannes J van Lieshout, David G Benditt

Introduction

Syncope is a syndrome defined as a transient, self-limited loss of consciousness. The underlying mechanism is a fall in systemic blood pressure resulting in transient global cerebral hypoperfusion. Loss of postural tone, often mentioned as an additional element, is in fact an inevitable consequence of loss of consciousness.

A sudden cessation of cerebral blood flow for only about 10 sec has been shown to be sufficient to cause complete loss of consciousness. Experience with tilt-table testing has taught us that a decrease in systolic blood pressure to 60 mmHg or less invariably leads to syncope. Furthermore, it has been estimated that a drop of as little as 20% in cerebral oxygen delivery is sufficient to cause unconsciousness.

In healthy young persons cerebral blood flow lies in the range of 50–60 mL per 100 g of brain tissue per minute, representing about 12–15% of resting cardiac output. A flow of this magnitude easily meets the minimum oxygen requirement to sustain consciousness (approximately 3.0–3.5 mL O_2/100 g tissue/min). However, the safety factor for oxygen delivery may be markedly impaired in older individuals or in those with diseases like diabetes mellitus or hypertension.

The integrity of a number of control mechanisms is crucial for maintaining adequate cerebral O_2 delivery.

- Arterial baroreceptor-induced adjustments of systemic vascular resistance, cardiac contractility and heart rate all act to modify systemic circulatory dynamics in order to protect cerebral blood flow.
- Intravascular volume regulation, incorporating renal and hormonal influences, helps to maintain central blood volume.
- Cerebrovascular autoregulation permits cerebral blood flow to be maintained over a relatively wide range of perfusion pressures.

Transient failure of protective mechanisms, or the additional effects of other factors such as vasodilator drugs, diuretics, dehydration or hemorrhage, any of which reduce systemic blood pressure below the autoregulatory range, may induce a syncopal episode. Risk of failure of normal protective compensatory mechanisms is greatest in older or ill patients.

This chapter discusses physiologic factors affecting the supply of blood to the brain, and discusses the clinical presentation of syncope, inasmuch as the clinical findings illuminate the pathophysiology of syncope. In addition, since failure of compensatory adjustments to orthostatic stress is thought to play an important role in the vast majority of patients with syncope (this concept forms the basis for the use of tilt testing in the evaluation of patients with syncope), a brief review of normal orthostatic blood pressure adjustment is provided first.

Goals

The goals of this chapter are to:
- review orthostatic blood pressure adjustment;
- discuss factors that may cause systemic hypotension and insufficient cerebral blood supply:
  low cardiac output
  low peripheral vascular resistance
  increased cerebrovascular resistance to blood flow; and
- discuss clinical presentation patterns of syncope.

Orthostatic blood pressure adjustment

On moving from the supine to the erect posture there is a large gravitational shift of blood away from the chest to the distensible venous capacitance system below the diaphragm (Fig. 2.1). This shift is estimated to total 0.5–1 L of thoracic blood, and largely occurs in the first 10 sec of standing. In addition, with prolonged standing, the high capillary transmural pressure in dependent parts of the body causes a filtration of protein-free fluid into the interstitial spaces. It is estimated that this results in a decrease of about 15–20% (700 mL) in plasma volume in 10 min in healthy humans. As a consequence of this gravitationally induced blood pooling and the superimposed decline in plasma volume, the return of venous blood to the heart is reduced. This results in a rapid diminution of cardiac filling pressure, and a decrease in stroke volume.

Despite the decreased cardiac output associated with movement to the upright posture, a fall in mean arterial pressure is prevented by a compensatory vasoconstriction of the resistance and the capacitance vessels in the splanchnic, musculocutaneous and renal vascular beds, and by an increase in heart rate. The vasoconstriction of systemic blood vessels is the key factor in the maintenance of arterial blood pressure in the upright posture. A pronounced heart rate increase on its own is insufficient to maintain cardiac output: the heart cannot pump blood that it does not receive.

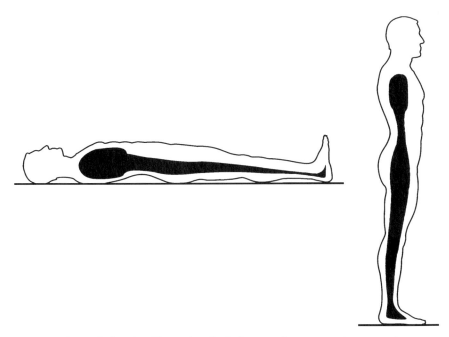

Fig. 2.1 Schematic drawing illustrating the influence of posture on intravascular volume. Note that in the supine figure (left), central blood volume (intrathoracic) is greater than when the figure is upright (right). The shift in blood volume to the lower extremities reduces venous return and cardiac output.

Rapid short-term compensation for the hemodynamic instability associated with orthostatic stress is mediated exclusively by neural pathways of the autonomic nervous system. During prolonged orthostatic stress, additional adjustments are mediated by the humoral limb of the neuroendocrine system (i.e., renin–angiotensin–aldosterone system and vasopressin).

The main sensory receptors involved in orthostatic neural reflex adjustments are the arterial mechanoreceptors (baroreceptors) located in the aortic arch and carotid sinuses (Fig. 2.2). Mechanoreceptors located in the heart and the lungs (cardiopulmonary receptors) are thought to play a minor role. Reflex activation of central sympathetic outflow to the systemic blood vessels can be reinforced by local mechanisms such as the venoarteriolar reflex and a myogenic response of the smooth blood vessels of resistance vessels in the dependent parts. The skeletal muscle pump and the "respiratory pump" play an important adjunctive role in the maintenance of arterial pressure in the upright posture by promoting venous return. Static increase in skeletal muscle tone of the lower limbs opposes orthostatic pooling of blood in limb veins. This latter mechanism occurs even in the absence of physical movement by the patient. However, any such movement (e.g., walking) would be expected to be of additional benefit by enhancing muscle pumping activity.

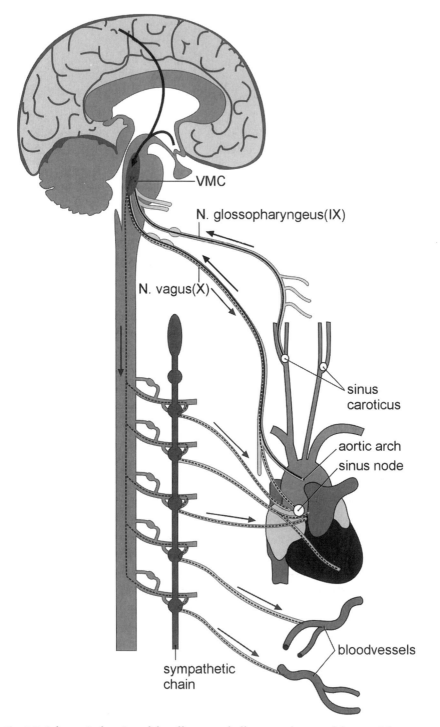

Fig. 2.2 Schematic drawing of the afferent and efferent pathways of the arterial baroreceptor reflex arc. Nerve fibres from the lungs and the heart (not shown) join the vagus nerve as cardiopulmonary afferents. VMC indicates vasomotor centres in the brainstem. (Revised after Timmers *et al. Ned Tijdschr Geneeskd* 2001; 145: 1413–1416.)

Factors that may cause insufficient cerebral blood supply

Pathophysiologic mechanisms

Cerebral perfusion pressure is largely dependent on systemic arterial pressure, which in turn depends on cardiac output and peripheral vascular resistance. Thus, anything that decreases either or both of these latter two factors will diminish systemic arterial pressure and cerebral perfusion pressure, and may thereby predispose to syncope. In addition to these two factors, any impairment to blood flow in the cerebrovascular vessels themselves, such as vasoconstriction, will also increase the chances of syncope.

A physiologic classification of mechanisms leading to reduced cerebral perfusion and syncope can be derived from the basic principles outlined above. A simple classification is summarized in Table 2.1, and each category is discussed briefly here.

Low peripheral resistance

Widespread and excessive vasodilatation may play a critical role in decreasing arterial pressure and thereby diminishing cerebral blood flow. In fact, this is the most frequent cause of cerebral hypoperfusion leading to syncope. Excessive vasodilatation is the main cause of fainting in the neural reflex syncopal disorders. These disorders refer to conditions in which neural reflexes which are normally useful in controlling the circulation (i.e., maintaining blood pressure) respond paradoxically. This results in a fall of systemic blood pressure due to vasodilatation and/or bradycardia (vasovagal reaction). In order to elicit this reflex a normal or functioning autonomic nervous system is necessary, in contrast to syncope due to orthostatic hypotension in patients with autonomic failure. Circumstances known to evoke neural reflex syncope are summarized in Table 2.1. It should be noted that the syncope induced by

Table 2.1 A physiologic approach to the causes of syncope.

Syncope primarily due to low peripheral resistance
Neural reflex syncope disorders such as vasovagal faint
Widespread cutaneous vasodilatation such as occurs during thermal stress
Vasodilator drugs
Autonomic neuropathies

Syncope primarily due to low cardiac output
Inadequate venous return—due either to excessive venous pooling or to low blood volume
Cardiac causes such as bradyarrhythmias, tachyarrhythmias, valvular heart disease and diminished left ventricular function

Syncope primarily due to increased resistance to cerebral blood flow
Low P_{CO_2} due to hyperventilation

increased intrathoracic pressure is mainly due to a decrease in venous return and only partially reflex mediated.

Impaired capacity to increase vascular resistance during standing is the principal cause of orthostatic hypotension and syncope in patients using vasoactive drugs, and in patients with various primary and secondary autonomic neuropathies.

Low cardiac output

With regard to maintenance of an adequate cardiac output, the most important physiologic determinant is the degree of venous filling. Venous return may become inadequate if there is an improper distribution of the circulating volume. An example is when blood is pooled excessively in lower parts of the body as occurs in some patients during movement to the upright posture. Obviously, a diminished total blood volume will also predispose to syncope, especially in conjunction with postural change. Cardiac output may also be impaired when the heart itself performs inadequately due to bradyarrhythmias, tachyarrhythmias, myocardial dysfunction or valvular heart disease.

The physiologic significance of changes in heart rate in the context of orthostatic stress merits consideration in this context. The relationship between heart rate (HR) and cardiac output (CO) is well known, namely:

$$CO = HR \times \text{stroke volume (SV)}$$

Although this equation is mathematically straightforward, it may be somewhat misleading in relation to understanding of physiologic control of blood pressure. This is because stroke volume is not usually independent of heart rate. Unless cardiac inflow (i.e., venous return) and cardiac contractility are enhanced, as occurs during whole-body exercise by the action of the leg muscle pump and high catecholamine levels, an increase in heart rate is accompanied by a decrease in stroke volume. Consequently, the increase in cardiac output is much less than expected. Conversely, if venous return is impaired (e.g., during venous pooling in the lower limbs), an increased heart rate may not compensate sufficiently.

Supraventricular tachycardia rarely causes syncope, except when rates are very high (usually > 200 beats/min) or in case of concomitant intrinsic structural cardiac disease (e.g., coronary artery disease, valvular stenosis). Ventricular tachycardia in contrast is a frequent cause of syncope or near-syncope. However, in this case it is the close association between ventricular tachycardia with underlying heart disease (especially left ventricular dysfunction) that is responsible. In the absence of structural heart disease, even relatively rapid ventricular tachycardias do not cause syncope.

As far as a low heart rate is concerned, the rate will have to decrease to well below 50 beats/min (and more often below 30 beats/min) for it to have a significant effect on cardiac output (in the absence of concomitant significant structural heart disease).

Increased resistance to cerebral blood flow

Cerebral hypoperfusion may also result from an abnormally high cerebral vascular resistance. Vasoconstriction, induced by low carbon dioxide tension due to hyperventilation, is probably the main cause, but sometimes the cause remains unknown. It has been suggested that this mechanism may contribute to the vasovagal faint in some patients, but the concept is controversial.

Clinical presentation patterns

Documented records of the hemodynamic and clinical events which precede a syncope under daily life circumstances are difficult to obtain. Consequently, voluntarily induced syncopal episodes under laboratory conditions have been studied. Two main approaches have been used. First, syncope may be induced instantaneously by using the combination of hyperventilation and straining. Secondly, the sequence of events during more gradually induced arterial hypotension can be studied by inducing vasovagal reactions in volunteers and patients using passive head-up tilt or subatmospheric pressure applied to the lower part of the body. In addition, observations in patients with cardiac syncope and patients with autonomic failure have contributed to the understanding of the events that are of importance for developing (pre)syncopal symptoms.

The "fainting lark": voluntary self-induced instantaneous syncope

The "fainting lark" (see also Chapter 15) is a maneuver that combines the effects of acute arterial hypotension due to the effect of gravity and raised intrathoracic pressure with cerebral vasoconstriction due to hypocapnia. The maneuver can be applied to induce almost instantaneous syncope in volunteers and may be used as a research tool. It consists of squatting in a full knee bend and overbreathing. The subject then stands up suddenly and performs a forced expiration against a closed glottis. The maneuver provokes a precipitous and deep fall in arterial pressure, and hyperventilation further reduces cerebral blood flow. The subject loses consciousness (Fig. 2.3).

Lempert and coworkers applied the "fainting lark" to study the sequence of events during syncope. Fifty-nine students aged 20–39 years volunteered for self-induction of syncope. Complete syncope was induced in 42 out of 59. Prodromal symptoms were short-lasting (< 5 sec), which is not surprising given the precipitous and deep fall in arterial pressure and cerebral blood flow induced by the "fainting lark" maneuver (Fig. 2.3). The loss of consciousness lasted 5–22 sec. Myoclonic jerks were observed in almost all of the 42 syncopal episodes. They occurred always after falling down and lasted 1–16 sec. During syncope, the EEG first shows large slow waves, signifying a profound disturbance of cortical function. When blood supply is not restored, these slow waves quite abruptly make way for a "flat" EEG, pointing to a complete cessation of function of cortical neurons. Unless blood flow is restored quickly, neurons

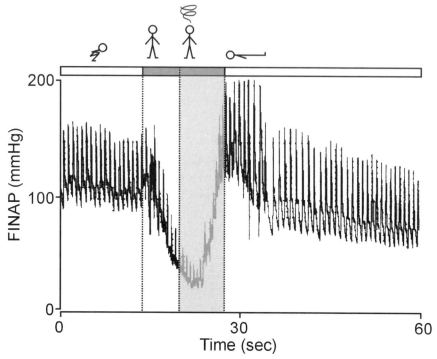

Fig. 2.3 Effect of the "fainting lark" on finger arterial pressure. For details about the procedure see text. Tracing obtained in a 54-year-old subject (WW). Note instantaneous, deep fall in arterial pressure. At the nadir of blood pressure the subject experienced a "black-out". Lying down, blood pressure recovers almost immediately and did overshoot. (Unpublished; by N. van Dijk and W. Wieling.)

will start dying, which is not reflected in any further EEG change. Provided that blood flow is restored before irretrievable damage has occurred, the EEG changes back to the normal state in reverse order. Myoclonic jerks occurring during the slow and flat stages are apparently from subcortical level.

Vasovagal syncope

Vasovagal syncope, also known as the common faint, is the most common of the neural reflex disorders (Table 2.2). The key circulatory alterations responsible for a vasovagal faint are vasodilatation (the vaso- component) and bradycardia (the vagal component).

Prodromal symptoms and signs are usually present in individuals experiencing spontaneous vasovagal syncope in daily life or induced vasovagal syncope under laboratory conditions. The first explanation for their occurrence is that patients usually have sufficient time to become aware of these feelings, as the fall in arterial pressure and cerebral perfusion pressure is usually more gradual in vasovagal syncope than in the fainting lark (compare Figs 2.3 &

Table 2.2 Circumstances known to evoke neural reflex syncope.

Vasovagal syncope
Emotionally induced
Orthostatic induced

Spontaneous carotid sinus syncope

Eyeball pressure

Gastrointestinal
Swallow syncope
Glossopharyngeal neuralgia
Esophageal stimulation
Gastrointestinal tract instrumentation
Rectal examination
Defecation syncope

Urogenital
(Post)micturition syncope
Urogenital tract instrumentation
Prostatic massage

Pulmonary
Airway instrumentation

Increased intrathoracic pressure
Cough and sneeze syncope
Wind instrument player's syncope
Weightlifter's syncope
Mess trick and fainting lark
Stretch syncope

Special situations
High altitude
Exercise-induced, diving

2.4). However, about one out of three individuals with vasovagal syncope (especially older patients) have little or no prodromal symptoms and the syncope essentially occurs instantaneously without any warning (usually because of a severe sudden-onset period of asystole).

A second reason for the occurrence of prodromal symptoms is the result of "autonomic activation" with symptoms and signs of sympathetic overactivity such as tachycardia, sweating and pallor, and later of parasympathetic overactivity such as bradycardia and nausea.

Prodromal symptoms sometimes occur minutes prior to the actual faint, but a period of only about 30 sec is probably more common. The patient begins to feel uncomfortable in an ill-defined way. This may be manifested by symptoms of epigastric discomfort and vague nausea, sweating and a desire to sit down or to leave the room. If these early warning symptoms

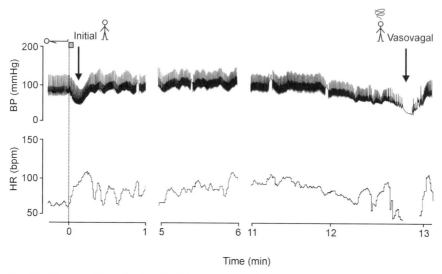

Fig. 2.4 Vasovagal fainting in a healthy 22-year-old male subject. Note normal initial heart rate and blood pressure response and marked increase in heart rate after 6 min standing. After 11–12 min standing, blood pressure and heart rate start to decrease to very low values during the faint; the heart rate tracing during the faint is interrupted by a period of asystole of 7 sec. On lying down, heart rate and blood pressure recover quickly, but blood pressure does not overshoot (with permission from Van Lieshout *et al.* 1991).

are ignored the disturbances increase and symptoms like lightheadedness, fatigue, blurred and fading vision, palpitations and tingling of the ears occur. The visual prodromal sensations are due to a reduction in blood supply to the retina. Since the eye, unlike the brain and brainstem, is not protected by the pressure-equalizing effects provided by the cerebrospinal fluid, the retina is exposed to the intraocular pressure and visual symptoms that result from collapse of retinal perfusion become manifest before consciousness is lost. This relationship has been studied in detail by exposure of subjects to large G-forces in whole-body centrifuges. Sensations begin with diminution of vision, gray-out (loss of color vision), which can then lead to "black-out". The moment of "black-out" occurs when the ischemic retina essentially ceases to function.

   Objective signs of an impending vasovagal faint are facial pallor, sweating, restlessness, yawning, sighing and hyperventilation and pupillary dilatation. The prodromal phase is most often associated with a relatively rapid heart rate (patient may note "palpitation" during this phase). With continuing hypotension the individual has difficulty in concentrating and becomes unaware of his surroundings. Some patients at this stage can still hear the conversation, but cannot move. When blood pressure falls further the patient loses consciousness and if standing falls to the floor. Severe bradycardia usually occurs late, immediately prior to the actual faint (Fig. 2.4).

The clinical picture during the actual faint resembles that of voluntarily induced syncope by the fainting lark. Myoclonic jerks, however, appear to be less common in spontaneous vasovagal syncope than in voluntarily induced syncope using the fainting lark. The duration of unconsciousness is almost always brief, usually lasting less than 5 min. Of additional importance in the overall clinical picture of vasovagal syncope are the postsyncopal findings, characterized by a persistence of pallor, nausea, weakness, sweating and oliguria, and a tendency toward recurrence of the reaction if the individual is returned to the upright posture. Fatigue, often lasting for several hours after the event, is also common (the latter observation led to the as yet controversial association of vasovagal physiology with certain forms of chronic fatigue syndrome).

Cardiac syncope

Syncope associated with heart block or with cardiac arrhythmias is usually characterized by sudden onset and absence of premonitory warning symptoms. However, in some patients with arrhythmias or heart block the onset is less abrupt, loss of consciousness need not be complete and sweating along with a sense of palpitation may occur. Nausea is rare in cardiac syncope. The syncopal episode may occur in either the erect or the prone posture. With cardiac arrest the patient is pulseless. Loss of consciousness usually ensues within 10 sec. It is reported that the loss of consciousness occurs more rapidly when the individual is standing than when he or she is recumbent. Prolonged asystole is complicated by myoclonic jerks and incontinence of urine. Recovery after termination of the arrhythmia is rapid with a sudden return of the pulse, flushing of the face and usually full orientation of the patient. The flush occurs during an overshoot in arterial pressure following the cardiac arrest.

Syncope due to orthostatic hypotension in patients with autonomic failure

Symptomatic orthostatic hypotension is the main problem in patients with autonomic failure. With a significant and persistent decrease in arterial pressure characteristic features occur. Symptoms include lightheadedness and blurring of vision. A neck ache radiating to the occipital region of the skull and to the shoulders (coathanger distribution) often precedes actual loss of consciousness. The postulated mechanism of this virtually unique symptom of postural hypotension is ischemia in continuously contracting postural muscles. Other symptoms suggesting impaired perfusion of muscle tissue are lower back and buttock ache or angina pectoris. Typically symptoms develop within minutes on standing or walking and resolve on lying down. The symptoms can be considered as prodromal symptoms and patients with autonomic failure quickly learn to use them as a warning sign that they must lie down to restore an adequate perfusion pressure. If the patient remains upright a gradual fading of consciousness occurs and the patient falls slowly to his or her knees. Sudden postural attacks may, however, also occur. Symptoms and signs of autonomic activation like sweating or a vagally induced bradycardia are absent in patients with autonomic failure.

Summary

The most important underlying mechanism of syncope is a transient pronounced fall in systemic blood pressure with cerebral hypoperfusion and loss of postural tone as its inevitable consequence. The most frequent cause is the neural reflex syncope disorders (such as a vasovagal faint). A low cardiac output, e.g., due to a heart block, can also cause syncope. Cardiac syncope is characterized by the suddenness of its onset and the lack of premonitory warning symptoms, thereby distinguishing it from the more slow onset of cerebral hypoxia and enhanced autonomic discharge in vasovagal syncope. Clinical presentation patterns of syncope often reveal the underlying pathophysiology involved.

Further reading

Van Lieshout JJ, Wieling W, Karemaker JM, Eckberg D. The vasovagal response. *Clin Sci* 1991; 81: 575–586.

Smit AAJ, Halliwill JR, Low PA, Wieling W. Topical review. Pathophysiological basis of orthostatic hypotension in autonomic failure. *J Physiol* 1999; 519: 1–10.

Hainsworth R. Syncope and fainting. In Mathias CJ, Bannister R. Autonomic failure. *A Textbook of Clinical Disorders of the Autonomic Nervous System*. Oxford, Oxford University Press 1999, pp. 429–436.

Lempert T, Bauer M, Schmidt D. Syncope: a videometric analysis of 56 episodes of transient cerebral hypoxia. *Ann Neurol* 1994; 36: 233–237.

Calkins H, Shyr Y, Frumin H, Schork A, Morady F. The value of clinical history in the differentiation of syncope due to ventricular tachycardia, atrioventricular block and neurocardiogenic syncope. *Am J Med* 1995; 98: 365–373.

Sutton R. Vasovagal syncope: prevalence and presentation. An algorithm of management in the aviation environment. *Eur Heart J* 1999; 1 (Suppl D): 109–113.

CHAPTER 3

Epidemiology and social costs

Rose Anne Kenny, Wishwa N Kapoor

Introduction

Syncope is a common problem. Forty per cent of us will experience syncope at least once in our lifetime. The majority of events are simple faints not requiring detailed investigation. Recurrent syncope, injurious events, or syncope in patients with structural heart disease or neurologic disorders require further attention.

Goals

The goals of this chapter are to provide an overview of:
- epidemiology of syncope including estimates of incidence and prevalence;
- prognosis;
- quality of life issues; and
- economic impact.

Certain of these issues are revisited in chapters addressing specific causes of syncope.

Epidemiology

The reported prevalence of syncope in the population varies depending on the group being studied. Thus, reports range widely: 15% of children before the age of 18; 25% of a military population aged 17–26; 16% and 19% in men and women aged 40–59 years; and up to 23% in a nursing home population of people greater than 70 years.

The highest frequency of syncope occurs in patients with cardiovascular comorbidity and older patients in institutional care settings. However, it should be noted that the quoted syncope prevalence figures for older people are undoubtedly an underestimate, given that up to 20% have amnesia for loss of consciousness and present with a fall rather than syncope.

Prognosis

The 1-year mortality of patients with cardiac syncope is consistently higher (ranging between 18 and 33%) than for patients with non-cardiac cause

(0–12%) or unexplained syncope (6%). One-year incidence of sudden death is 24% in patients with a cardiac cause compared with 3% in the other two groups. Although patients with cardiac syncope have higher mortality rates compared with those of non-cardiac or unknown causes, patients with cardiac causes do not appear to exhibit a higher mortality when compared with matched controls who have similar degrees of heart disease. The presence and severity of structural heart disease are the most important predictors of mortality. It may reasonably be expected that syncope patients with multiple comorbidities, and thereby multiple potential causes for syncope, will have an even higher mortality.

Excess mortality rates in syncope patients with ventricular tachyarrhytmias are highest in those with severe ventricular dysfunction (Table 3.1). One-year mortality in patients with syncope due to cardiac arrhythmias increases exponentially from 4% (no other risk factor) to 80% in patients with three or more risk factors—this algorithm incorporating risk factors is useful for risk stratification.

Structural heart disease is a major risk factor for sudden death and overall mortality in patients with syncope (Table 3.1). The association of syncope with aortic stenosis has been long recognized as having an average survival without valve replacement of 2 years. Similarly, in hypertrophic cardiomyopathy, the combination of young age, syncope at diagnosis, severe dyspnea and a family history of sudden death best predict sudden death. In arrhythmogenic right ventricular dysplasia, patients with syncope or symptomatic ventricular tachycardia have a similarly poor prognosis. Patients with ventricular tachyarrhythmias have higher rates of mortality and sudden death but the excess mortality rates depend on underlying heart disease; patients with severe ventricular dysfunction have the worst prognosis. Some of the cardiac causes of syncope do not appear to be associated with increased mortality. These include most types of supraventricular tachycardias and sick sinus syndrome.

A number of subgroups of patients can be identified who have an excellent prognosis (Table 3.1). Certain of these include young healthy individuals without heart disease and normal electrocardiogram (ECG), neurally mediated syndromes, orthostatic hypotension (the mortality rates of patients with orthostatic hypotension depend on the causes of this disorder), and syncope of unknown cause (5% 1st-year mortality in patients with unexplained syncope).

Recurrences

One third of patients have recurrences of syncope at 3 years of follow-up. The majority of these recurrences occur within the first 2 years (but presumably continue into the future in untreated individuals). Predictors of recurrence of syncope include having had recurrent syncope at the time of presentation, age less than 45 years or a psychiatric diagnosis. After positive tilt-table testing, patients with more than six syncopal spells have a risk of recurrence of more than 50% over 2 years.

Recurrences are not proven to be associated with increased mortality or sudden death rates, but patients with recurrent syncope have a poor functional status similar to patients with other chronic diseases.

Table 3.1 Syncope: prognostic stratification.

---

1   Cardiac disease—general
Age ≥ 45 years, history of congestive heart failure, history of ventricular arrhythmias and abnormal ECG (other than non-specific ST changes)
Cardiac arrhythmias are a cause of syncope or death (or cardiac death) within 1 year of follow-up in 4% without any of these risk factors increasing to 80% in patients with three or more factors

2   Structural heart disease—specific conditions with poor prognosis
Aortic stenosis
In syncopal patients without valve replacement, the average survival is 2 years

Hypertrophic cardiomyopathy
The combination of young age, syncope at diagnosis, severe dyspnea and a family history of sudden death best predict sudden death

Arrhythmogenic right ventricular dysplasia
Patients with syncope or symptomatic ventricular tachycardia have poor prognosis

Ventricular tachyarrhythmias
Patients have higher rates of mortality and sudden death but the excess mortality rates depend on underlying heart disease; patients with severe ventricular dysfunction have the worst prognosis

3   Structural heart disease—specific conditions with better prognosis
Young healthy individuals (less than 45 years of age) without heart disease and normal ECG
There is no evidence that these patients have an increased mortality risk. Most have neurally mediated or unexplained syncope

Neurally mediated reflex syncope
The mortality at follow-up is near 0%. Most of these patients have normal hearts

Orthostatic hypotension
The mortality rates of patients with orthostatic hypotension depend on the causes of this disorder and comorbid illnesses

Supraventricular tachycardias and sick sinus syndrome
These cardiac causes of syncope are not associated with increased mortality

Syncope of unknown cause (after thorough evaluation)
First-year mortality is 5%. Although the mortality is largely due to underlying comorbidity, such patients continue to be at risk for physical injury, and may encounter employment and lifestyle restrictions

---

Physical injury

Syncope may result in injury to the patient or to others. This may occur when a patient is driving or working in an environment where injury might result from loss of postural control. Major morbidity such as fractures and motor vehicle accidents are reported in 6% of patients, and minor injury such as laceration and bruises in 29%. There is no data on the risk of injury to others.

Recurrent syncope is associated with fractures and soft tissue injury in at least 12% of patients.

Quality of life

Functional impairment in syncope patients is similar to chronic illnesses such as rheumatoid arthritis, low back pain and psychiatric disorders. Impairment is evident in domains such as mobility, usual activities, self-care, pain and dis-comfort, and anxiety and depression. There is a marked negative relationship between the frequency of spells and overall perception of health.

Economic implications

Patients with syncope are often admitted to hospital and undergo expensive and repeated investigations, many of which do not provide a definite diagno-sis. Despite the advent of newer diagnostic tests (e.g., tilt testing, wider use of electrophysiologic testing, loop ECG monitoring) the management of syncope remains disparate and unstructured in most centers (see Chapter 7). Patients often undergo a great number of tests at considerable cost.

Estimated hospital costs are in excess of 10 billion US dollars per year. This is undoubtedly an underestimate because many patients with syncope are not admitted to hospital, and the costs of their care may not be adequately captured.

Summary

Syncope occurs frequently in the population, and recurrences are common. The evaluation of syncope remains largely unstructured in most centers. The result is frequent use of ineffective testing strategies at considerable cost to the health care system.

Further reading

Lewis DA, Dhala A. Syncope in the pediatric patient. The cardiologist's perspective. *Pediatr Clin North Am* 1999; 46(2): 205–219.

Lipsitz LA, Wei JY, Rowe JW. Syncope in an elderly, institutionalized population: prevalence, incidence, and associated risk. *Q J Med* 1985; 55(216): 45–54.

Oh JH, Hanusa BH, Kapoor WN. Do symptoms predict cardiac arrhythmias and mortal-ity in patients with syncope? *Arch Intern Med* 1999; 159(4): 375–380.

The Multicentre Post Infarction Group. Risk stratification and survival after myocardial infarction. *N Engl J Med* 1983; 309: 331–336.

Martin TP, Hanusa BH, Kapoor WN. Risk stratification of patients with syncope. *Ann Emerg Med* 1997; 29(4): 459–466.

Rose MS, Koshman ML, Spreng S, Sheldon R. The relationship between health-related quality of life and frequency of spells in patients with syncope. *J Clin Epidemiol* 2000; 53(12): 1209–1216.

Kapoor WN, Peterson J, Wieand HS, Karpf M. Diagnostic and prognostic implications of recurrences in patients with syncope. *Am J Med* 1987; 83(4): 700–708.

Soteriades ES, Evans JC, Larson MG, Chen MH, Chen L, Benjamin EJ *et al.* Incidence and prognosis of syncope. *N Engl J Med* 2002; 347(12): 878–885.

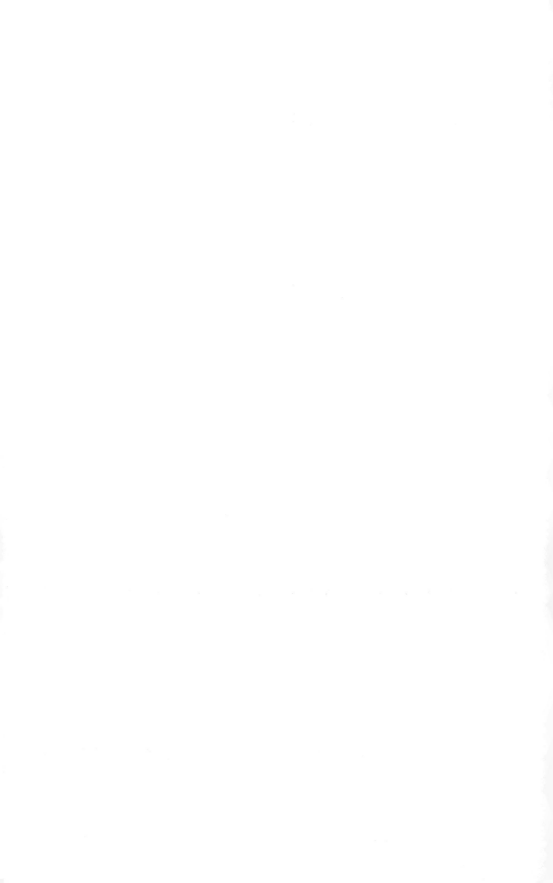

Section two:
Syncope evaluation strategy

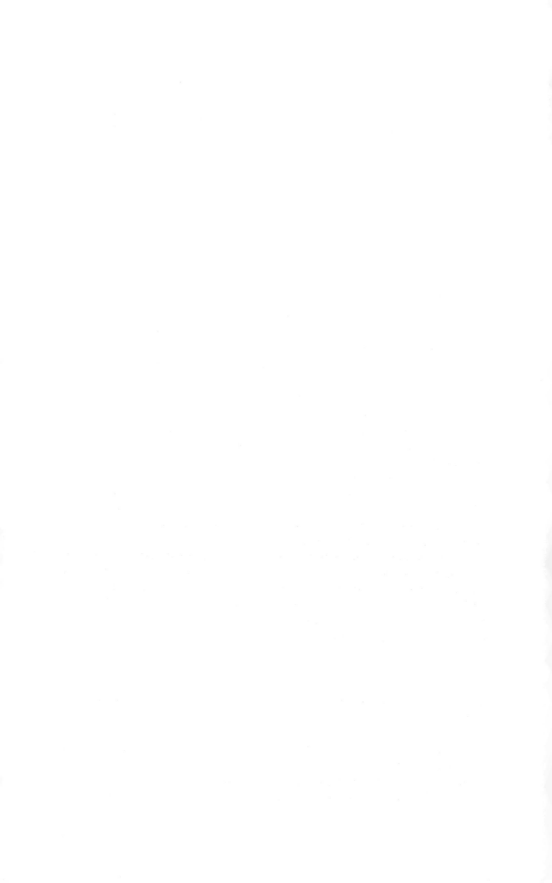

CHAPTER 4

Overview of recommended diagnostic strategies

Richard Sutton, Michele Brignole

Introduction

Many conditions may present as transient loss of consciousness. Syncope is one of the most common and clinically important of these. However, apart from determining whether the loss of consciousness was due to true syncope (see Chapter 1), it is crucial to determine the basis of syncope in each patient. In this regard, the cause or causes of syncope in an individual may be multiple. Further, even in those cases where a single cause appears to be to blame, multiple comorbidities may interact, thereby increasing susceptibility to fainting (e.g., abrupt movement to upright posture in a patient with diabetic neuropathy).

The starting point for the evaluation of syncope is a careful history and physical examination including orthostatic blood pressure measurements. These aspects of the initial evaluation are discussed in more detail in subsequent chapters. Techniques for appropriate and complete medical history-taking in syncope patients (reviewed in Chapter 5) merit particular attention given the importance of the history in providing a presumptive diagnosis, and directing subsequent diagnostic testing (Table 4.1).

In most young patients without heart disease, and with typical symptom presentation (Table 4.1), a definite diagnosis of neurally mediated vasovagal syncope can often be made without any further testing. Except for this case, a 12-lead electrocardiogram (ECG) should be usually part of the general evaluation of patients (Table 4.2). This basic assessment will be defined as the "initial evaluation" (see Chapter 5 for greater detail).

Goals

The aim of this chapter is to provide a succinct overview of a reasonable strategy for assessment of patients with suspected syncope. Three issues will be addressed:
- approach to the patient in whom the basis for syncope seems certain after "initial evaluation";
- approach when the etiology is uncertain; and
- approach when the diagnosis remains unknown after the initial evaluation.

Table 4.1 Clinical features suggestive of specific causes.

Symptom or finding	Possible cause
After sudden unexpected unpleasant sight, sound, or smell	Vasovagal
Prolonged standing at attention or crowded, warm places	Vasovagal or autonomic failure
Nausea, vomiting associated with syncope	Vasovagal
Within 1 hour of a meal	Postprandial (autonomic failure)
After exertion	Vasovagal or autonomic failure
Syncope with throat or facial pain	Neuralgia (glossopharyngeal or trigeminal neuralgia)
With head rotation, pressure on carotid sinus	Spontaneous carotid sinus syncope (as in tumors, shaving, tight collars)
Within seconds to minutes upon active standing	Orthostatic hypotension
Temporal relationship with start of medication or changes of dosage	Drug induced
During exertion, or supine	Cardiac syncope
Preceded by palpitation	Tachyarrhythmia
Family history of sudden death	Long QT syndrome, Brugada syndrome, right ventricular dysplasia, hypertrophic cardiomyopathy
In course of a migraine attack	Migraine
Associated with vertigo, dysarthria, diplopia	Brainstem transient ischemic attack (TIA)
With arm exercise	Subclavian steal
Differences in blood pressure or pulse in the two arms	Subclavian steal or aortic dissection
Confusion after attack for more than 5 minutes	Seizure (see Chapters 12 and 17)
Tonic–clonic movements, automatism, tongue biting, blue face, epileptic aura	Seizure (see Chapters 12 and 17)
Frequent attack with somatic complaints, no organic heart disease	Psychiatric illness

The initial evaluation (see also Chapter 5)

Three key questions need to be considered during the initial evaluation.
- Is loss of consciousness attributable to syncope or not?
- Is heart disease present or absent?
- Are there important clinical features in the history that suggest the diagnosis? Differentiating "true" syncope from other "non-syncopal" conditions associated with real or apparent transient loss of consciousness is generally the first diagnostic challenge. This decision, which usually relies on interpretation of a detailed medical history along with reports from eye-witnesses, markedly

Table 4.2 ECG abnormalities suggesting an arrhythmic syncope.

Bifascicular block (defined as either left bundle branch block or right bundle branch block
    combined with left anterior or left posterior fascicular block)
Other intraventricular conduction abnormalities (QRS duration ≥ 0.12 sec)
Mobitz I 2nd degree atrioventricular block
Asymptomatic sinus bradycardia (< 50 bpm) or sinoatrial block
Pre-excited QRS complexes
Prolonged QT interval
Right bundle branch block pattern with ST-elevation in leads V1–V3 (Brugada syndrome)
Negative T waves in right precordial leads, epsilon waves and ventricular late potentials
    suggestive of arrhythmogenic right ventricular dysplasia
Q waves suggesting myocardial infarction

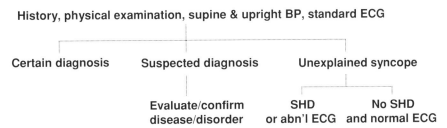

Fig. 4.1 This schematic illustrates a recommended diagnostic strategy for the diagnostic evaluation of syncope patients. The first step is the initial evaluation (see Chapter 5). Thereafter, patients can be categorized as having a "certain diagnosis", or a "suspected diagnosis" (i.e., likely but not absolutely sure in the eyes of the physician), or "unexplained". See text for further details. SHD, structural heart disease; BP, blood pressure.

influences the subsequent diagnostic testing strategy. Historical features outlined below and in Chapter 5 must be carefully considered in each patient prior to coming to this judgement.

The diagnostic outcome from the "initial evaluation" may be a "certain" diagnosis, a "suspected" diagnosis, or "no known" diagnosis (Fig. 4.1). In each instance, the experience of the physician plays a major role in ascertaining the presumed diagnosis, and in judging whether further testing is desirable.

In the case of the diagnosis being "certain" after the "initial evaluation", further testing may be unnecessary depending on the physician's confidence in the "certainty" of the assessment. In the case of a "suspected" diagnosis, the subsequent direction for confirmatory testing is established by having come to at least a presumption of the cause. The latter paves the way for an efficient and cost-effective evaluation. When the initial evaluation is unable to provide any clue as to the diagnosis (here termed as "unexplained syncope") the strategy for subsequent diagnostic steps depends on the frequency and severity of the episodes and the nature of any underlying heart disease.

Certain diagnosis

On occasion, the initial evaluation may lead to a relatively "certain" diagnosis based on symptoms, signs or ECG findings. Under such circumstances, no further evaluation of the disease or disorder may be needed and treatment, if any, can be planned. The following provides examples of such situations.

- Vasovagal syncope is diagnosed if precipitating events such as fear, severe pain, emotional distress, instrumentation or prolonged standing are associated with typical prodromal symptoms in patients without evidence of underlying heart disease.
- Situational syncope is diagnosed if syncope occurs during or immediately after certain circumstances, such as urination, defecation, coughing or swallowing.
- Orthostatic syncope is diagnosed when there is documentation of orthostatic hypotension associated with syncope or presyncope. Orthostatic blood pressure measurements are recommended after 5 min of lying supine, followed by each minute, or more often, after standing for 3 min. Measurements may be continued longer if blood pressure is still falling at 3 min. If the patient does not tolerate standing for this period, the lowest systolic blood pressure during the upright posture should be recorded. A decrease in systolic blood pressure (20 mmHg) or a decrease of systolic blood pressure to < 90 mmHg is defined as orthostatic hypotension regardless of whether or not symptoms occur.
- Cardiac ischemia-related syncope is diagnosed when symptoms are present with ECG evidence of acute ischemia with or without myocardial infarction. However, whether the syncope was due to a neurally mediated reflex (i.e., bradycardia and vasodilatation) or the result of an ischemia-induced cardiac arrhythmia may require further assessment.
- Arrhythmia-related syncope is only rarely "diagnosed" by the 12-lead ECG during the initial evaluation. More often, an ambulatory long-term ECG recording is needed. However, the 12-lead ECG may provide sufficient evidence when there is:
    (i)   sustained sinus bradycardia < 40 beats/min (other than during sleep) or repetitive asystolic pauses (i.e., sinoatrial block, sinus pauses) > 3 sec in duration in the absence of negatively chronotropic medications;
    (ii) Mobitz II 2nd or 3rd degree atrioventricular block;
    (iii) alternating left and right bundle branch block in ischemic heart disease;
    (iv) rapid paroxysmal supraventricular tachycardia or ventricular tachycardia; or
    (v)   pacemaker malfunction with cardiac pauses.

Suspected diagnosis

More commonly, the initial evaluation leads to a "suspected" diagnosis, which needs to be confirmed by directed testing. Thus, in the case of suspected vaso-vagal faint, a head-up tilt-table test would be the next step. Thereafter, depending on how convincing the result is (i.e., did it reproduce patient symptoms?) further steps might be needed. The reader is referred to Chapters 8–13 for details regarding appropriate diagnostic procedures.

Unexplained diagnosis

The strategy for subsequent assessment of patients in whom the initial evaluation resulted in "no known" diagnosis varies according to the severity and frequency of the episodes and the presence or absence of heart disease. Apart from the prognostic importance of the presence of heart disease, its absence excludes a cardiac cause of syncope with few exceptions. In a recent study, heart disease was an independent predictor of cardiac cause of syncope, with a sensitivity of 95% and a specificity of 45%; by contrast, the absence of heart disease allowed exclusion of a cardiac cause of syncope in 97% of patients.

For patients without structural heart disease and who have a normal ECG (Fig. 4.2), evaluation for neurally mediated syncope is recommended for those with recurrent or severe syncope. The tests for neurally mediated syncope primarily consist of tilt testing and carotid massage. The majority of patients with single or rare episodes in this category probably have neurally mediated syncope. Since treatment is generally not recommended in this group of patients, close follow-up without evaluation is recommended. For patients with signs of autonomic failure or neurologic disease, a specific diagnosis should be made. An additional consideration in patients without structural heart disease, with a normal ECG, and with many faints, is psychiatric illness. Psychiatric assessment is especially recommended for patients with frequent "syncope" (actually pseudo-syncope, see Chapter 17) recurrences in conjunction with multiple other somatic complaints and medical concern for stress, anxiety and possibly other psychiatric disorders.

In patients with structural heart disease or who have an abnormal ECG (Fig. 4.2), cardiac evaluation consisting of echocardiography, stress testing and tests for arrhythmia detection such as prolonged ambulatory ECG (AECG) monitoring (including use of implantable loop recorders, ILRs) or electrophysiologic study are recommended. If cardiac evaluation does not show evidence of arrhythmia as a cause of syncope, evaluation for neurally mediated reflex syndromes is recommended in those with recurrent or severe syncope.

For patients with palpitations associated with syncope, AECG monitoring and echocardiography are recommended. ILR monitoring is a valuable tool and should be used in patients with recurrent unexplained syncope whose symptoms are suggestive of arrhythmic syncope. In patients with chest pain suggestive of ischemia before or after loss of consciousness, stress testing

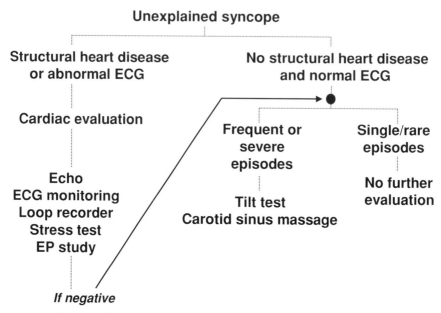

Fig. 4.2 Schematic illustrating the basic evaluation strategy for patients in whom the diagnosis remains "unexplained" after the steps in Fig. 4.1 have been completed. See text for details.

and echocardiography are recommended. AECG monitoring may have additional value in certain cases. Similarly, for patients with syncope during or after effort, echocardiography and stress testing are recommended as first evaluation steps.

Summary

The medical history provides the cornerstone for diagnosing the cause of syncope. A detailed history needs to be obtained in each case, often incorporating the observations of witnesses. Thereafter, the experienced physician can judge whether additional diagnostic testing is needed. The European Society of Cardiology Syncope Task Force statement provides useful guidance for appropriate diagnostic testing for syncope patients. The subsequent chapters of this handbook provide practical clinical advice based on the guideline document.

Further reading

Alboni P, Brignole M, Menozzi C et al. The diagnostic value of history in patients with syncope with or without heart disease. *J Am Coll Cardiol* 2001; 37: 1921–1928.

Brignole M, Alboni P, Benditt D et al. Guidelines on management (diagnosis and treatment) of syncope. *Eur Heart J* 2001; 22: 1256–1306.

Moya A, Brignole M, Menozzi C *et al*. Mechanism of syncope in patients with isolated syncope and in patients with tilt-positive syncope. *Circulation* 2001; 104: 1261–1267.

Brignole M, Menozzi C, Moya A *et al*. The mechanism of syncope in patients with bundle branch block and negative electrophysiologic test. *Circulation* 2001, 104: 2045–2050.

Menozzi C, Brignole M, Garcia-Civera R *et al*. Mechanism of syncope in patients with heart disease and negative electrophysiologic test. *Circulation* 2002; 105; 2741–2745.

Benditt DG, Brignole M. Syncope: is a diagnosis a diagnosis? *J Am Coll Cardiol* 2003; 41: 791–794.

Initial evaluation of the syncope patient

Part 1: Medical history and basic laboratory assessment

Antonio Raviele, Paolo Alboni, Richard Sutton, Rose Anne Kenny

Introduction

The initial diagnostic approach to patients with syncope comprises a detailed medical history (incorporating documentation of eye-witness accounts), a thorough physical examination (including supine and standing blood pressure measurements), and 12-lead electrocardiogram (ECG). Basic laboratory tests (measurement of electrolytes, blood counts, and tests of renal function and glucose level) are usually not indicated in the initial evaluation of patients with syncope. As a rule, such tests have a low diagnostic yield (2–3%) and are recommended only if a loss of circulating volume, severe anemia, marked dehydration, or a syncope-like disorder with a metabolic cause is suspected.

The history and physical examination are the core of the work-up for patients with syncope. Alone, they permit the cause of loss of consciousness to be established in approximately 45% of cases, as a metanalysis of data from six population-based studies has shown (Table 5.1).

Goals

This part of the chapter provides:
- a review of the elements essential to the initial diagnostic evaluation of syncope patients; and
- a technique for obtaining a detailed medical history for evaluation of syncope.

When taking the medical history the first important issue is differentiating true syncope from several other conditions that resemble syncope (i.e., may produce or appear to produce "loss of consciousness"), but that are not due to a generalized reduction in cerebral blood flow. Examples of such conditions include seizures, drop attacks and somatization disorders (see Chapters 12, 13 & 14, Part 5).

Table 5.1 Causes of syncope found by history and physical examination or electrocardiography.

Study	Patients (*n*)	Diagnosis by history and physical examination (*n* (%))	Diagnosis by ECG (*n* (%))
Kapoor	433	140 (32)	30 (7)
Ben-Chetrit	101	33 (33)	11 (11)
Martin	170	90 (53)	2 (1)
Eagle and Black	100	52 (52)	
Silverstein	108	42 (38)	
Day	198	147 (74)	4 (2)
All studies	1110	504 (45)	47 (5)

Adapted from Linzer M *et al. Ann Intern Med* 1997; 126: 989–996.

Distinguishing syncope from a generalized seizure (epilepsy) may be particularly difficult using medical history and bystander observations alone (see also Chapter 17, Table 17.4). In brief, features that are indicative of epilepsy include:
- tonic–clonic movements that are usually prolonged and coincident with the onset of loss of consciousness;
- hemilateral clonic movements;
- clear automatisms such as chewing or lip smacking or frothing at the mouth (partial seizure);
- tongue biting, blue face;
- aura such as unusual or distinctive smell before the event; and
- prolonged confusion and aching muscles after the event.

In patients with syncope, the jerky muscular movements are usually of short duration (< 15 sec), always start after the loss of consciousness, and are typically asynchronous and limited in scope (so called "myoclonic").

The most important features of the history that must be taken into consideration when evaluating patients with syncope are reported in Table 5.2.

Taking the medical history in syncope patients: a method

Obtaining a detailed medical history is the first step in the assessment of the cause or causes of syncope. If the history-taking is careful and thorough, the story provided by the patient (and witnesses) will often reveal the most likely cause of the faint, and will provide a means of guiding an efficient and cost-effective subsequent evaluation to confirm the clinical suspicion.

A classification of the principal causes of syncopal episodes has been provided earlier in this book. This classification provides a means of organizing one's thoughts when initiating the medical history-taking in a new patient, and it should be kept in mind throughout the process. In this section we

Table 5.2 Important historical features.

Questions about circumstances just prior to attack
Position (supine, sitting or standing)
Activity (rest, change in posture, during or after exercise, during or immediately after urination, defecation, cough or swallowing)
Predisposing factors (e.g., crowded or warm places, prolonged standing, postprandial period) and precipitating events (e.g., fear, intense pain, neck movements)

Questions about onset of attack
Nausea, vomiting, abdominal discomfort, feeling of cold, sweating, aura, pain in neck or shoulders, blurred vision, chest pain, palpitations

Questions about attack (eye-witness)
Way of falling (slumping or kneeling over), skin color (pallor, cyanosis, flushing), duration of loss of consciousness, breathing pattern (snoring), movements (tonic, clonic, tonic–clonic or minimal myoclonus, automatism) and their duration, onset of movement in relation to fall, tongue biting

Questions about end of attack
Nausea, vomiting, feeling of cold, sweating, confusion, muscle aches, skin color, injury, chest pain, palpitations, urinary or fecal incontinence

Questions about background
Family history of sudden death, congenital arrhythmogenic heart disease
Previous cardiac disease
Neurologic history (Parkinsonism, epilepsy, narcolepsy)
Metabolic disorders (diabetes etc.)
Medication (antihypertensive, antianginal, antidepressant agent, antiarrhythmic, diuretics and QT prolonging agents)
(In the case of recurrent syncope) Information on recurrences such as the time from the first syncopal episode and the number of spells

---

highlight certain of the most important clinical features often associated with various causes of syncope. In order to take advantage of this information, the details surrounding syncope events must be documented in considerable detail by the careful history-taker. Thereafter, we provide a basis upon which the historical features may be used to suggest a specific cause for the faint. However, history-taking is very user experience-dependent, and even in the best circumstances the sensitivity of the process is not established. False positives and false negatives are bound to occur. Consequently, confirmatory testing (albeit focused by virtue of having considered the historical findings) is more often than not essential in order to establish a confident diagnosis.

Important components of the medical history in syncope

Before beginning the history-taking it is important to determine whether the patient can give an accurate account of events. This limitation particularly applies to older patients who may have cognitive impairment. In such cases it is crucial that an informant in regular contact with the patient should attend the consultation, and be interviewed as part of the history-taking process. Indeed, whenever possible, try to secure a witness account.

General features

In order to characterize the patient's faints, it is helpful to have the patient focus on the most recent event. After a thorough description is obtained, turn the patient's attention to the next most recent episode. Be demanding of details. Witnesses can be very valuable in filling in items that the patient may not recall. Obtain details on as many events as you feel is necessary to assess the symptoms. Are there features common to all or at least some of the episodes?

In some patients multiple causes may be responsible for symptoms. These may be identified or at least suggested by the medical history. Pay attention to the presence of comorbidities. Comorbidities may act synergistically (e.g., diabetic neuropathy and drug-induced orthostasis), or they may act independently thereby resulting in more than one "cause" for the faint.

Among the factors of importance from a general perspective are: Frequency of episodes? Over what period of time? Duration of loss of consciousness (this is often inaccurately reported, or at least is hard to substantiate)? Associated presyncope or "dizziness" (or other similar complaint)? History of falls or unexplained accidents? Nature of physical injuries sustained if any? Any common thread with regard to time of onset?

Characterizing situations in which syncope tends to occur: is there a pattern?

Position: Supine, sitting or standing?

Activity: At rest (supine, upright)? With change in posture? During or after exercise? During or immediately after voiding? During or after defecation, cough or swallowing?

Circumstances: Occurs in crowded or warm places? During prolonged standing? During the postprandial period? Associated with fear, intense pain or being emotionally upset? In conjunction with abrupt neck movements (particularly looking upward)?

Identifying prodromal symptoms

Are symptoms associated with nausea, vomiting, feeling of cold, sweating, visual aura, pain in neck or shoulders, blurred vision, palpitations?

Documenting eye-witness observations during the faint

Describe the manner in which the fall occurred (e.g., abrupt fall with possibility of injury, purposeful avoidance of injury); skin color changes associated with the faint; duration of loss of consciousness; breathing pattern; physical movements (e.g., tonic-clonic or myoclonic movements); incontinence; tongue biting.

Symptoms noticed after the event

Confusion, palpitations, duration of symptoms, headache, nausea, vomiting, sweating, feeling of cold, muscle aches, skin color, injury, chest pain.

Characterizing patient risk for syncope recurrence and/or life-threatening consequences

Family history

Is there a family history of sudden death? Known genetically transmitted arrhythmogenic states (e.g., long QT syndrome, arrhythmogenic ventricular dysplasia)? Familial predisposition to syncope (fainting, "black-outs", "spells", etc.)? Migraine history?

Fainter's medical history

Is there any evidence of structural cardiac disease (e.g., prior infarction, valvular heart disease, congenital conditions, previous cardiac surgery, etc.)? Neurologic conditions (e.g., Parkinsonism, epilepsy, migraine)? Metabolic/intoxication disorders (e.g., diabetes, alcoholism)? Drug abuse (e.g., cocaine, diuretics)?

Prescribed medication predisposing to syncope

Is the patient taking drugs known to predispose to syncope such as antihypertensives, antianginal drugs, antidepressant agents, antiarrhythmics, diuretics and QT prolonging agents? Has there been any recent dosing change? Have any new drugs been added that might produce an undesirable interaction?

Indicators from the history suggestive of specific causes

Table 5.3 provides a short list of historical findings that suggest specific causes of syncope. The reader is referred to chapters dealing with each of these diagnoses for greater detail.

Additional elements of the initial evaluation

Physical findings that are useful in diagnosing syncope are orthostatic hypotension, cardiovascular signs and neurologic signs (less often). Orthostatic hypotension has been found in 8% of patients with syncope. Important cardiovascular findings include differences in blood pressure in each arm, pathologic cardiac and vascular murmurs, signs of pulmonary embolism, aortic stenosis, idiopathic hypertrophic cardiomopathy, myxomas and aortic dissection. Signs of focal neurologic lesions, such as hemiparesis, dysarthria, diplopia and vertigo, or signs of Parkinsonism are suggestive of (but not diagnostic of) a neurologic cause of impairment of consciousness. Such patients warrant a neurologic evaluation. In general, however, neurologic disease is a very rare cause of syncope.

Table 5.3 Clinical elements considered diagnostic of a specific cause of syncope.

Vasovagal syncope
Association of precipitating events (fear, severe pain, emotional distress, instrumentation, prolonged standing) with typical prodromal symptoms (nausea, vomiting, sweating, feeling of cold, tiredness)

Situational syncope
Occurrence of syncope during or immediately after urination, defecation, cough or swallowing

Orthostatic syncope
Documentation of orthostatic hypotension (decrease in systolic blood pressure (20 mmHg or to < 90 mmHg) associated with reproduction of symptoms (syncope or presyncope)

Ischemia-related syncope
Simultaneous presence of symptoms and ECG signs of acute ischemia with or without myocardial infarction

Arrhythmia-related syncope
Sinus bradycardia < 40 beats/min or repetitive sinoatrial blocks or sinus pauses > 3 sec; Mobitz II 2nd or 3rd degree atrioventricular block; alternating left and right bundle branch block; rapid paroxysmal supraventricular tachycardia or ventricular tachycardia; pacemaker malfunction with cardiac pauses

The 12-lead ECG identifies with certainty a specific (arrhythmic) cause of syncope in only a small percentage of cases (5%). However, from time to time the 12-lead ECG documents findings such as a Q wave, left ventricular hypertrophy, a prolonged QT interval or ventricular pre-excitation that may suggest or indicate the presence of organic heart disease, and thereby provides a basis for proceeding with further testing.

When the initial evaluation (history, physical examination and 12-lead ECG) is diagnostic, the work-up can be stopped, and if indicated, treatment may be planned and started. On the other hand, when the initial evaluation is only suggestive, or is non-diagnostic for a specific cause, the investigation must be continued. The situations in which the initial evaluation is considered diagnostic are reported in Table 5.3. Other investigations beyond the initial evaluation are discussed elsewhere in this book (see Chapter 4 and Chapters 8–13).

Even when inconclusive, the initial evaluation is often useful because it may reveal abnormalities that suggest the possible cause of syncope, thus guiding the subsequent evaluation strategy. Clinical and ECG findings that are clues to specific diagnoses are reported in Tables 5.3 and 5.4, respectively. Carotid sinus massage is a recommended diagnostic step in all patients (especially older individuals). For patients with a suggested diagnosis after the initial evaluation, specific "confirmatory" testing is often warranted in order to solidify the suspected diagnosis, or "rule out" the diagnosis. Such testing may also

Table 5.4 ECG findings supporting a cardiac arrhythmia basis for syncope*.

Sinus bradycardia < 40 beats/min
Sinoatrial blocks or sinus pauses > 3 sec
Mobitz II or 3rd degree atrioventricular block
Alternating left and right bundle branch block
Rapid paroxysmal supraventricular tachycardia or ventricular tachycardia
Pacemaker malfunction with cardiac pauses
Long QT syndrome, Brugada syndrome
Pre-excitation (Wolff–Parkinson–White) syndrome

* The nature of the causal arrhythmia requires further evaluation (see Chapter 14, Part 3) which may encompass ambulatory ECG monitoring (see Chapter 8), and electrophysiologic testing (see Chapter 10).

aid in the planning of treatment. Tilt-table testing is an example of a "confirmatory" test which is often used when the diagnosis of a vasovagal faint is suspected, but the presentation was not classical. Tilt testing is most valuable in individuals without evident structural heart disease.

When the results of the initial evaluation are completely non-diagnostic, the patient may be considered to have "unexplained syncope". Decisions about further testing should be based on an assessment of the patient's risk factors. In patients with structural heart disease and/or abnormal ECG, additional cardiac evaluation is indicated to exclude a mechanical or arrhythmic cause of syncope. In patients without structural heart disease and having a normal ECG, an evaluation for a neurally mediated reflex origin of syncope will need to be revisited because the majority of these patients have a vasovagal syncope (i.e., high pretest probability). However, patients with single or rare spells and without clinical evidence of organic heart disease may not need an especially invasive evaluation because they have a low risk of syncopal recurrences and a good overall prognosis.

Summary

This chapter focuses on the initial evaluation of the syncope patient. The medical history is the key in every case. Reports from witnesses should also be sought and recorded. The 12-lead ECG and perhaps an echocardiogram are reasonably included in the initial evaluation. In many cases, no further evaluation is needed after the initial evaluation. However, even when inconclusive, this stage of the syncope assessment sets the stage for efficient and cost-effective selection of subsequent confirmatory studies.

Further reading

Hoefnagels WAJ, Padberg GW, Overweg J *et al.* Transient loss of consciousness: the value of the history for distinguishing seizure from syncope. *J Neurol* 1991; 238: 39–43.

Martin GJ, Adams SL, Martin HG *et al*. Prospective evaluation of syncope. *Ann Emerg Med* 1984; 13: 499–504.

Alboni P, Brignole M, Menozzi C *et al*. The diagnostic value of history in patients with syncope with or without heart disease. *J Am Coll Cardiol* 2001; 37: 1921–1928.

Calkins H, Shyr Y, Frumin H, Schork A, Morady F. The value of clinical history in the differentiation of syncope due to ventricular tachycardia, atrioventricular block and neurocardiogenic syncope. *Am J Med* 1995; 98: 365–373.

Oh JH, Hanusa BH, Kapoor WN. Do symptoms predict cardiac arrhythmias and mortality in patients with syncope? *Arch Intern Med* 1999; 159: 375–380.

Linzer M, Yang EH, Estes III M *et al*. Diagnosing syncope. Part 1: Value of history, physical examination, and electrocardiography. *Ann Intern Med* 1997; 126: 989–996.

Kapoor WH. Syncope. *N Engl J Med* 2000; 343: 1856–1862.

Brignole M, Alboni P, Benditt D *et al*. Guidelines on management (diagnosis and treatment) of syncope. *Eur Heart J* 2001; 22: 1256–1306.

CHAPTER 5

Initial evaluation of the syncope patient

Part 2: Role of defined questionnaire for diagnosis of syncope and other forms of transient loss of consciousness

Robert Sheldon

Introduction

There are numerous causes of transient total loss of consciousness (TLOC), and their prevalence depends on the population that is studied. Although some of the less common causes of TLOC are potentially life-threatening (e.g., certain cardiac arrhythmias), and some such as epilepsy have substantial implications for lifestyle issues such as driving, most patients faint for benign reasons that do not pose an immediate threat to their life (although injury may occur). All the dangerous causes of TLOC and many of the benign causes of syncope merit treatment; treating patients successfully begins with an accurate diagnosis.

The accurate and efficient diagnostic work-up of syndromes of TLOC can be difficult. Although many patients pose no diagnostic problems, not infrequently clinicians must consider a number of possible etiologies. One of the problems has been a reluctance to trust the history of unconsciousness as an important source of information. This has led to reliance on investigative tools that measure structural and functional aspects of the central nervous system; ischemic, electrical and structural aspects of the cardiovascular system; and various endocrinologic disorders. Most of these have a very limited diagnostic yield for unselected patients with a history of TLOC, most are expensive or invasive or both, and most continue to be used early in the diagnostic cascade. Are there other tests that might have a higher diagnostic yield?

Goals

The goals of this part of the chapter are to:
- identify limitations of current diagnostic strategies for evaluating TLOC; and

• introduce the concept of a predefined questionnaire as a means of enhancing diagnostic assessment of TLOC, and in particular of distinguishing syncope from seizures.

Limitations of tilt tests and implantable loop recorders (ILRs)

Two popular diagnostic tools are tilt-table tests and implantable loop recorders. Tilt tests are thought to reproduce some aspect of the disturbed physiology that underlies the syndrome or collection of syndromes of vasovagal syncope. Tilt tests have been enormously useful in the study of neurally mediated syncope. They have provided a diagnosis in most patients with otherwise unexplained syncope, have been useful tools in the study of its physiology, and have provided uniformly diagnosed populations for natural history studies and clinical trials. Implantable loop recorders record the electrocardiogram (ECG) during syncope, and are therefore a screen for arrhythmic causes of syncope and for neurally mediated syncope syndromes associated with transient, autonomically mediated bradycardias. They have established the diagnostic outcomes of patients at elevated risk for arrhythmic syncope, and have provided valuable information about the heart rate of patients with probable neurally mediated syncope during their spells.

Head-up tilt tests, although seemingly simple, are precariously balanced on a number of important variables. Carefully controlled studies have shown that the likelihood of positive studies in both syncope patients and control subjects depends on a number of factors (see also Chapters 9 & 14, Part 1) including:
• angle of the head-up tilt-table;
• duration of head-up tilt;
• whether a drug challenge is used, and the type and dose of drug challenge;
• number of head-up iterations during the tilt test;
• volume status of the subject; and
• subject age.

There is a variable correlation between the symptoms provoked by tilt testing and the subject's clinical symptoms, and widely variable and usually unvalidated hemodynamic criteria. Importantly, there is no gold standard population against which the test has been validated. This is important because different tilt test protocols appear to identify patient populations that do not overlap completely. Tilt test protocols, each with adequate specificities, are positive in populations that do not overlap. If they both have reasonable albeit imperfect accuracies, then which one is true? Can we diagnose patients with a test that appears to only diagnose a subset of truly positive patients? Finally, there appears to be an intractable trade-off between sensitivity and specificity. No single tilt test protocol now appears to function at a reliably high level.

The implantable loop recorder (ILR) also has potential problems. It is a passive tool that relies on the patient having another syncopal spell—unless one is willing to accept a surrogate rhythm which has not caused syncope (e.g., non-sustained ventricular tachycardia) as a working "diagnosis". While waiting for syncope recurrence may be tolerable to some, it is not optimal for evaluation of patients with high likelihood of a potentially fatal causes of syncope. Therefore, ILR use may be best restricted to patients with "benign" causes of syncope (although the benign nature of the cause cannot be readily predicted ahead of time). Further, an ILR is invasive and its cost-effectiveness depends upon its sensitivity and the consequences of a diagnosis. Therefore the loop recorder is unlikely to find a niche in diagnosing patients with dangerous causes of syncope. On the other hand, in the setting of more benign causes of syncope it may detect many periods of non-diagnostic sinus rhythm since most of these are vasovagal syncope in which the "classic" (but not necessarily common) finding of a long asystolic pause is not present.

Can we take a better history?

Considerations such as the limitations of diagnostic tools discussed above suggest that we need to reassess the usefulness of the medical history in TLOC patients. Clinical educators have long taught that symptoms such as generalized convulsions denote a diagnosis of epilepsy, while associated nausea and vomiting denote a diagnosis of vasovagal syncope. Although symptoms such as seizure-like activity, tongue biting and physical trauma are often used to diagnose a seizure disorder, this practice has been based upon anecdotal accretion rather than evidence. Furthermore, the recognition of "convulsive syncope" has added to the difficulties of diagnosis. Many have felt that there is little to be learned from the symptoms associated with TLOC, since unconsciousness patients by definition do not remember their symptoms. However quantitative histories and diagnostic scores are well known in other fields; they are known to improve diagnostic accuracy; and there are known quantitative differences in the histories among patients with different causes of TLOC.

Quantitative histories

Both Calkins *et al.* and Alboni *et al.* reported that patients with different causes of syncope, such as ventricular tachycardia, complete heart block and vasovagal syncope, have highly significant differences in the symptoms that accompany loss of consciousness. However, these differences in symptoms generally provide clinicians with a sense of the differences among the groups, rather than providing them with simple tools that can be used in decision-making. These problems can be overcome with a quantitative analysis of the symptoms, expressed as a diagnostic point score. These point scores are likely to be quite useful. The reliability of the diagnosis of the first loss of consciousness is surprisingly low, but this can be improved with preset simple diagnostic criteria. This suggests that a structured questionnaire, if based on firm quantitative evidence, might be helpful in the assessment of the patient with TLOC.

The syncope symptom study

We hypothesized that evidence-based diagnostic criteria could distinguish between syncope and seizures as causes of transient loss of consciousness. To test this we performed the Syncope Symptom Study. A uniform questionnaire was administered to 671 patients who were referred to three academic centres in Canada and Wales for assessment of TLOC. We first studied patients with securely defined diagnoses based upon conventionally accepted objective tests. Then we compared their responses to identify the historical features that most accurately correlated with their diagnoses. The causes of TLOC were known satisfactorily in 539 patients and included complex partial epilepsy, primary generalized epilepsy, tilt-positive vasovagal syncope, ventricular tachycardia, and other diagnoses such as complete heart block and supraventricular tachycardias. The point score based on symptoms alone correctly classified 94% of patients, diagnosing seizures with 94% sensitivity and 94% specificity. Therefore a simple point score of historical features distinguished syncope from seizures with very high sensitivity and specificity.

We have recently developed two similar questionnaires. The first of these was designed for assessing patients with syncope in the setting of structural heart disease. The diagnostic dilemma that is faced with this population is that 20–40% of patients have ventricular tachycardia as a cause of their syncope, and if recurrent this can be fatal. Some patients have complete heart block, and many have vasovagal syncope. Current investigations such as electrophysiologic testing have variable sensitivities and specificities, and may be inadequate. For example, invasive electrophysiologic testing is only 50% and 70% sensitive for ventricular tachycardia in the settings of idiopathic dilated cardiomyopathy and old inferior myocardial infarction. We have developed a brief quantitative questionnaire that is 90% sensitive and 90% specific for distinguishing between ventricular tachycardia and vasovagal syncope, and have found that about two-thirds of patients with negative electrophysiologic studies and negative tilt tests resemble patients with ventricular tachycardia. The second questionnaire, also brief, has similar accuracy in the population of patients with syncope and apparently structurally normal hearts.

Conclusion

These three questionnaires, if validated in other populations, may prove useful in managing patients with TLOC. Although they are not meant to be the sole source of diagnostic decisions, they may prove helpful to the clinician in the initial diagnostic assessment. They will provide inclusion criteria for population-based studies and clinical trials, permit a quantitative link among the various causes of vasovagal syncope, and allow us to examine the physiology of syncope in subgroups of patients who share common diagnostic criteria. If accepted by clinicians, they may significantly reduce the time, expense and inaccuracy of the assessment of patients with total transient loss of consciousness.

Further reading

Van Donselaar CA, Geerts AT, Meulstee J, Habbema JDF, Staal A. Reliability of the diagnosis of a first seizure. *Neurology* 1989; 39: 267–271.

Calkins H, Shyr Y, Frumin H, Schork A, Morady. The value of the clinical history in the differentiation of syncope due to ventricular tachycardia, atrioventricular block, and neurocardiogenic syncope. *Am J Med* 1995; 98: 365–373.

Linzer M, Yang EH, Estes III NA *et al*. Diagnosing syncope. Part I. Value of history, physical examination, and electrocardiography. *Ann Int Med* 1997; 126: 989–996.

Alboni P, Brignole M, Menozzi C *et al*. Diagnostic value of history in patients with syncope with or without heart disease. *J Am Coll Cardiol* 2001; 37: 1921–1928.

Sheldon R, Rose S, Ritchie D *et al*. Historical criteria that distinguish syncope from seizures. *J Am Coll Cardiol* 2002; 40: 142–148.

CHAPTER 6

Which syncope patients should be evaluated and treated in hospital, and which can be managed as outpatients?

David G Benditt

Introduction

Syncope by definition implies that the patient has suffered a transient period of loss of consciousness, and by virtue of the loss of consciousness had lost the capability to maintain postural tone for at least a short period of time. In such a circumstance, the outcome could include risk of personal injury, as well potential risks to others. However, from the perspective of whether the patient needs hospitalization for the syncope, the driving force is most often uncertainty regarding immediate mortality risk, and to a lesser extent the issue of whether certain treatments require hospital monitoring for safe initiation.

Goals

The goals of this chapter are to:
- identify those risk factors which if present would favor hospitalizing a patient for the syncope evaluation;
- classify conditions in which hospitalization is not needed; and
- summarize treatment choices which necessitate hospitalization.

When is hospitalization advised?

The admission decision can be considered with two different objectives: for diagnosis or for therapy. For patients with syncope in whom the etiology remains unknown after the initial baseline evaluation, risk stratification can be used to determine if hospitalization is prudent (see later). In instances when the etiology of syncope has been diagnosed after the initial clinical evaluation, the hospitalization decision depends in part on the immediate risk posed to the patient by the underlying problem and in part on the treatment proposed. Thus, for example, patients with syncope accompanying an acute myocardial infarction, or pulmonary embolism, or torsades de pointes ventricular tachycardia should be admitted. Patients with dehydration due to excess diuretic therapy usually do not need admission. Similarly, in terms of therapy to be initiated, patients needing pacemakers or implantable cardioverter defibrillators (ICDs) will be admitted, possibly along with those in whom initiation of certain types of antiarrhythmic drugs is contemplated. On the other hand, for patients being treated with salt and volume, or physical maneuvers like tilt training or leg crossing, an outpatient initiation is usually adequate.

Hospitalization recommendations

Strongly recommended

Several prognostic markers assist in identifying syncope patients who should be considered for in-hospital evaluation. The presence of underlying structural heart disease and abnormalities of the baseline ECG are important markers for cardiac syncope. An important, but less frequent, prognostic marker is the family history of sudden death, since certain malignant ventricular arrhythmias can have a genetic basis (e.g., long QT syndrome (LQTS), Brugada syndrome, familial cardiomyopathies). These entities are discussed in more detail in later chapters (see Chapter 14, Part 3). Table 6.1 summarizes those conditions in which hospitalization for syncope assessment is strongly recommended. Tables 6.2 and 6.3 provide details of ECG findings, and specific clinical scenarios that favor hospitalization.

Table 6.1 When to hospitalize a patient with syncope for diagnosis.

Strongly recommended for diagnosis
Suspected or known significant heart disease
ECG abnormalities suggestive of arrhythmic syncope (Table 6.2)
Syncope occurring during exercise (Table 6.3)
Syncope causing severe injury
Family history of sudden death

Occasionally may need to be admitted
Patients with or without heart disease but with:
   sudden onset of palpitations shortly before syncope
   syncope in supine position
Patients with minimal or mild heart disease when there is high suspicion for cardiac syncope
Suspected pacemaker or ICD problem

Table 6.2 ECG findings supporting hospital admission for diagnosis.

Acute myocardial infarction
Acute pulmonary embolism
Complete or high-grade atrioventricular block
Long QT syndrome
Brugada syndrome
Wolff–Parkinson–White syndrome with atrial fibrillation and rapid ventricular response

Table 6.3 Causes of syncope during exercise.

Critical coronary artery disease
Severe valvular/subvalvular disease
Congenital coronary artery anomaly
High-grade atrioventricular block
Long QT (LQTS, KvLQT1)

Table 6.4 When to hospitalize a patient with syncope for treatment.

Strongly recommended
Cardiac arrhythmias as cause: drug initiation, probable radio frequency ablation (RFA), pacemaker/ICD
Ischemic cause: revascularization, drug initiation, exercise testing
Neurally mediated: when pacemaker proposed, after significant injury/accident
Severe orthostatic hypotension
Associated focal neurologic abnormality: stroke, hemorrhage
Orthopedic injury/fracture

Hospitalization desirable on case-by-case basis

These situations generally involve patients in whom the risk of death is thought to be low, and there is low likelihood of a near-term recurrence precipitating injury or harm to the public health (Table 6.4).

When is it safe not to hospitalize?

For patients with isolated or rare syncopal episodes, in whom there is no evidence of structural heart disease and who have a normal baseline ECG, the probability is high that the event was of neurally mediated origin (see also Chapter 14, Part 1). The risk of having a life-threatening cardiac syncope is low. These patients have a good prognosis in terms of survival and generally their evaluation can be completed entirely on an outpatient basis. Nevertheless, cautionary advice regarding driving, occupations and/or avocation restrictions should be provided until such time as one is confident that the susceptibility to fainting has been suppressed.

Table 6.5 Low-risk scenarios favoring outpatient evaluation.

Isolated or rare syncope without:
- cardiac disease or significant ECG abnormality
- pacemaker or ICD present
- worrisome physical injury
- public health hazard in compliant patient
History typical of vasovagal or situational faint
History suggestive of syncope mimic (see Chapter 17)

Patients with neurally mediated reflex faints (especially vasovagal faints, and with the possible exception of carotid sinus syndrome) generally do not need specific treatment apart from counseling and the general measures discussed in Chapter 14, Part 1. If treatment is needed because of recurrences, it can usually be initiated on an ambulatory basis.

Table 6.5 summarizes those clinical findings associated with low risk of severe injury and/or death in a syncope patient. These individuals represent good candidates for outpatient evaluation and treatment.

Summary

The decision to hospitalize a patient with syncope for diagnostic evaluation and/or initiation of therapy depends primarily on the short-term mortality risk to the patient. In older individuals, the short-term morbidity risk also plays a role (i.e., fracture risk if syncope recurs in the elderly). Additional concerns relate to public well-being, such as might be at risk if a non-compliant fainter resumes driving a commercial vehicle or piloting an aircraft.

There are no convincing data regarding risk of death or injury during the out-of-hospital evaluation of syncope patients. However, if the risk stratification provided here is used, the chances of an adverse outcome during the evaluation and treatment initiation phase should be remote.

Further reading

Brignole M, Alboni P, Benditt DG *et al*. Guidelines on management (diagnosis and treatment) of syncope. *Eur Heart J* 2001; 22: 1256–1306.

CHAPTER 7

Organizing management of syncope in the hospital and clinic (the syncope unit)

Rose Anne Kenny, Michele Brignole

Introduction

Inasmuch as syncope is a common symptom—experienced by 15% of persons under 18 years and up to 23% of older nursing home residents—it is important to consider optimizing strategies for the management of these patients. The strategy selected will inevitably differ from place to place depending on patient volume, available resources and the expertise of medical personnel. However, ultimately, an organized structure will offer more cost-effective care.

Goals

The goals of this chapter are to:
- outline possible health care delivery models for syncope management;
- review current status of the organization of syncope care; and
- summarize the Newcastle experience to illustrate the value of a multidisciplinary approach to the organized management of syncope patients.

General features of the syncope care delivery organization

There is no single syncope care delivery model suitable for all environments. The following offers a list of some of the more important features to consider when establishing such an organization.
- The model of care delivery should be that which is most appropriate to existing practice and will maximize resources and local expertise while ensuring implementation of published practice guidelines.
- Models of care delivery will vary from a single "one site–one stop" syncope facility to a wider-based multifaceted practice where a number of specialists are involved in syncope management. The management strategy should be agreed upon and practised by all practitioners (encompassing a range of specialities) involved in syncope management.

- The age range and symptom characteristics of patients appropriate for syncope investigation should be determined in advance. Some facilities are prepared to evaluate both pediatric and adult syncope patients, while others limit practice to adult or pediatric cases.
- Potential referral sources should be taken into consideration. Referral can be directly from family practitioners, from the accident and emergency department, from hospital admissions, and from patients in institutional settings. The scope of referral source has implications for resources and skill mix.
- In a single dedicated facility the skill mix will depend on the specialty designated to take a lead in the development of the facility. There are existing models where cardiologists (commonly with an interest in cardiac pacing and electrophysiology), neurologists (commonly with an interest in autonomic disorders and/or epilepsy), general physicians, and geriatricians (with an interest in age-related cardiology or falls) have each led syncope facilities. There is no evidence for superiority of any model.
- One factor which will influence the skill mix (i.e., the types of professionals/expertise required to staff the facility) is the extent to which screening of referrals occurs prior to presentation at the facility. If referrals hail directly from the community and/or from the accident and emergency department, a broader skill mix is required. Under these circumstances, other differential diagnoses such as epilepsy, neurodegenerative disorders, metabolic disorders and falls are more likely to be referred.
- It is essential to establish a mechanism through which regular communication can be established with all stakeholders (i.e., patients, referring physicians, hospital/clinic management, consultant physicians, nurses and other allied medical professionals) in order to ensure an ongoing consensus for and understanding of proposed management strategies. This includes the implications of, and implementation of published guidelines. Among the medical profession stakeholders it is important to consider staff members in cardiology, the accident and emergency department, neurology department, general medicine service, orthopedic surgery, geriatric medicine, psychiatry and ear, nose and throat (ENT) department.

Need for coordinating the syncope evaluation

Emerging data suggests that up to 20% of cardiovascular syncope in older patients (over 70 years) presents as non-accidental falls. There is also evidence from the "falls" literature that multifactorial intervention which includes cardiovascular interventions (treatment of orthostatic hypotension, carotid sinus hypersensitivity, arrhythmias and vasovagal susceptibility) significantly reduces subsequent falls in fallers with recurrent episodes—even if these are accidental falls. This has enormous implications for the volume of patients seen. It requires access to, or incorporation of, assessments and interventions for other common comorbid risk factors such as gait and balance instability, cerebrovascular disease, home hazard modifications, etc. An example of the scope of this issue is illustrated in a study from Newcastle. Forty-four per cent of accident and emergency attendees over 65 years came to the syncope evaluation unit because of a fall or syncopal event. Of these patients, 35% had accidental falls, 25% were patients who had cognitive impairment or dementia (therefore a clear distinction between falls/syncope was often not possible), 22% had a medical explanation for the event, and 18% had unexplained falls.

Present syncope management (diagnosis and treatment) situation

Syncope is a common symptom in the community and in emergency medicine. For example, in the UK, syncope and collapse (International Classification of Diagnoses code 10) are the sixth commonest reason for admission of adults aged over 65 years to acute medical hospital beds. Given that half of all emergency admissions are over 65 years, this constitutes a large volume of activity. The average length of stay for these admissions is 5–17 days—emphasizing the diversity of syncope management strategies and availability of existing investigations.

Currently, strategies for assessment for syncope vary widely among physicians and among hospitals and clinics. More often than not, the evaluation and treatment of syncope is haphazard and unstratified. The result is a broad and largely inexplicable variance from center to center in the frequency with which various diagnostic tests are applied, in the distribution of apparent attributable causes of syncope arrived at by attending clinicians, and in the proportion of syncope patients in which the diagnosis remains unexplained. One example of this is pacing rates for carotid sinus syndrome which vary even within countries from 1 to 25% of implants, depending on whether carotid sinus hypersensitivity is systematically assessed in the investigation profile. Another example is the prevalence of syncope that remains unexplained. This varies from 10 to 70%.

Assuming the status quo of the syncope evaluation is maintained, diagnostic and treatment effectiveness is unlikely to improve substantially. Even implementation of the published syncope management guidelines is likely to be diverse, uneven in application, and of uncertain benefit. It is the ESC Syncope Task Force's view that a cohesive, structured care pathway—delivered either within a single syncope facility or as a more multifaceted service—is now timely. In this manner, considerable improvement in diagnostic yield and cost-effectiveness (i.e., cost per reliable diagnosis) can be achieved by focusing skills and following well defined up-to-date diagnostic guidelines.

Newcastle syncope management unit model

The service model adopted by the Newcastle group is a multidisciplinary approach to referrals with syncope or falls. All patients attend the same facility (with access to cardiovascular equipment, investigations and trained staff) but are investigated by a geriatrician or cardiovascular physician according to the dominant symptom cited in referral correspondence—falls or syncope. Recently, this group showed that activity at the acute hospital at which the day case syncope evaluation unit was based, experienced 6116 fewer bed-days during the course of one year for the ICD code 10 categories comprising syncope and collapse compared to peer teaching hospitals in the UK. This reduction translated into a significant saving in emergency hospital costs (about 4 million euros or US dollars). The savings were attributed to a combination of factors—reduced readmission rates, rapid access to day case facilities for accident and emergency staff and community physicians, and implementation of effective targeted treatment strategies for syncope and falls.

Professional skill mix for the syncope evaluation facility

It is probably not appropriate to be dogmatic regarding the training needs of personnel responsible for a dedicated syncope facility. These skills will depend on the predetermined requirements of local professional bodies, the level of screening evaluation provided prior to referral, and the nature of the patient population typically encountered in a given setting. In general, experience and training in key components of cardiology, neurology and geriatric medicine which are pertinent to the assessment and diagnosis of syncope, in addition to access to other specialisms such as psychiatry, physiotherapy, occupational therapy, ENT and clinical psychology are recommended.

Staff responsible for the clinical management of the facility should be conversant with the various appropriate diagnostic and treatment guidelines. The principal guidelines are as follows: "Guidelines on management (diagnosis and treatment) of syncope", "Guidelines for the prevention of falls in older persons", and "Clinical guidelines for treatment and practical tools for aiding epilepsy management" (see Further reading for citations). A structured approach to the management of syncope also expedites clinical audit, patient information systems, service developments and continuous professional training.

Equipment

Core equipment for the syncope evaluation facility includes surface electrocardiogram (ECG) recording, phasic blood pressure (BP) monitoring, tilt-table testing equipment, external and implantable ECG loop recorder systems, and 24-h ambulatory BP, 24-h ambulatory ECG and autonomic function testing. The facility should also have access to intracardiac electrophysiologic testing, stress testing, cardiac imaging, CT and/or MRI/head scans and electroencephalography.

Setting

The majority of syncope patients can be investigated as outpatients or day cases.

Indications for hospital admission (see Chapter 6 as well) and investigation are those cases in which syncope occurs in association with one or more of the following:
- significant heart disease (particularly critical valvular or subvavular aortic stenosis, severe coronary artery disease);
- suspected serious cardiac arrhythmias (e.g., long QT syndromes, Brugada syndrome);
- physical exercise;
- severe injury; or
- family history of sudden death.

Summary

In summary, the role of a local integrated syncope service is to set standards for, and optimize the effectiveness of, the evaluation and treatment of syncope patients at a given center. This is best accomplished by a multidisciplinary approach, and should be in keeping with appropriate guidelines such as those established by the objectives of the European Society of Cardiology Syncope Task Force Guidelines. The standards should consider, at a minimum, the following issues.
- The diagnostic criteria for causes of syncope.
- The preferred approach to the diagnostic work-up in subgroups of patients with syncope.
- Risk stratification of the patient with syncope.
- Treatments to prevent syncopal recurrences.

When establishing a newly structured service, current experience suggests that careful audit of the syncope unit activity and performance will rapidly justify the initial resource allocation and requests for additional funding, fuel further service development, and provide a legitimate magnet for increasing patient referrals.

Further reading

Brignole M, Alboni P, Benditt D *et al*. Guidelines on management (diagnosis and treatment) of syncope. *Eur Heart J* 2001; 22(15): 1256–1306.

Guideline for the prevention of falls in older persons. American Geriatrics Society, British Geriatrics Society, and American Academy of Orthopaedic Surgeons Panel on Falls Prevention. *J Am Geriatr Soc* 2001; 49(5): 664–672.

Royal College of Physicians. Adults with poorly controlled epilepsy: Clinical guidelines for treatment and practical tools for aiding epilepsy management. July 1997. ISBN 186016062 X. Code 15113002.

Kenny RA, O'Shea D, Walker HF. Impact of a dedicated syncope and falls facility for older adults on emergency beds. *Age Aging* 2002; 31: 272–275.

Kenny RA, Richardson DA, Steen N *et al*. Carotid sinus syndrome: a modifiable risk factor for nonaccidental falls in older adults (SAFE PACE). *J Am Coll Cardiol* 2001 November 1; 38(5): 1491–1496.

Shaw FE, Bond J, Richardson DA *et al.* Multifactorial intervention after a fall in older people with cognitive impairment and dementia presenting to the accident and emergency department. *Br Med J* 2003; 326: 73–77.

Section three:
Guide to selection of diagnostic procedures

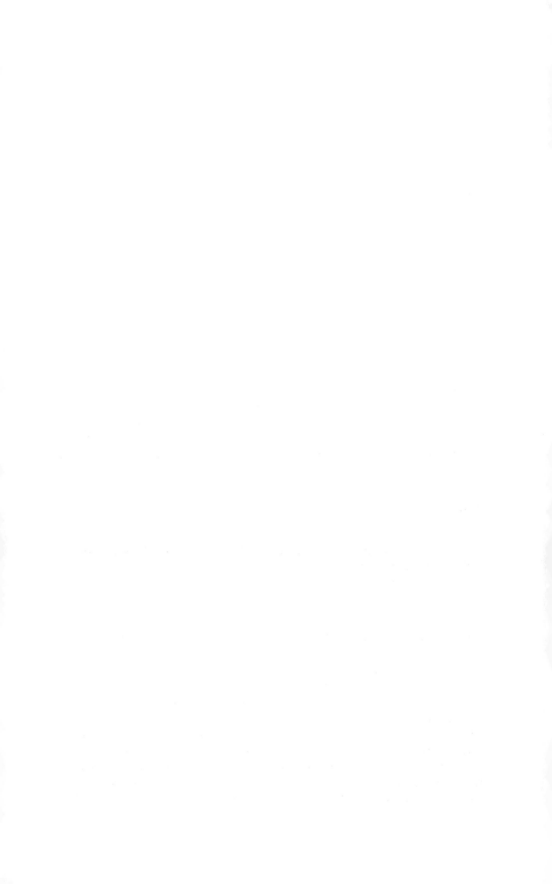

CHAPTER 8

Ambulatory electrocardiographic (AECG) monitoring for evaluation of syncope

Adam P Fitzpatrick

Introduction

Syncope is often infrequent. Consequently it is difficult to document spontaneous symptoms by a diagnostic investigation. Electrocardiographic (ECG) monitoring is one of the most important tools used to establish a basis for syncope by determining a symptom–ECG correlation. However, ECG monitoring is constrained by technologic limitations.

Goals

The goals of this chapter are to:
- review currently available ambulatory ECG (AECG) systems applicable to the evaluation of syncope patients; and
- provide recommendations regarding AECG systems for various circumstances.

Ambulatory electrocardiographic monitoring options

Holter monitoring

AECG monitoring for evaluation of patients with syncope is most often undertaken using an external 24-h cassette tape-recorder (Holter monitor). The recorder is connected to the patient via external wiring and conventional adhesive ECG patches. The advantages of this technology are several; it is noninvasive, there is beat-to-beat complete acquisition of the heart rhythm over the period of monitoring (as long as the electrode patches remain secure), the recording device costs are low, and there is relatively high recording fidelity over short time periods. However, the limitations of this technology are that a recurrence of presenting symptoms is unlikely to occur during monitoring, that patients may not tolerate adhesive surface electrodes for more than a few days, and that electrodes may not remain adherent throughout monitoring, or during an event. The vast majority of patients with syncope have a symptom frequency measured in weeks, months or years, but not days. Symptom–ECG correlation is rarely achieved with Holter monitoring for syncope. The diagnostic yield is variably reported to be between 6 and 20%, but may in fact be much less (see later).

Conventional AECG monitoring can be problematic in that an asymptomatic arrhythmia detected by Holter is often used to make a diagnosis by inference, but without symptom–ECG correlation. Further, there is potential for symptoms to be inappropriately minimized if Holter monitoring fails to yield any evidence of an arrhythmia. This is particularly likely because many physicians may not understand that given the low likelihood of recording a spontaneous event during the limited Holter recording period (usually 24 or 48 h), Holter monitoring generally offers a very low diagnostic yield in the syncope evaluation. Our studies and others indicate that the true diagnostic yield of Holter ECG monitoring in syncope is about 1%.

Holter monitoring in syncope is inexpensive in terms of set-up cost, but since the diagnostic yield is low, the test is expensive in terms of cost per diagnosis. This is especially the case if a very large number of tapes must be recorded to yield a symptom–ECG correlation. In this regard, it may be reasonable to avoid unnecessary analysis of "asymptomatic" tapes, and simply analyze "symptomatic" tapes. However, while such a strategy may reduce cost in some respects, it nevertheless requires provision of very large numbers of tape-recorders to service the need, greatly increasing another aspect of cost.

Given the rarity with which an AECG–syncope correlation can be obtained by Holter monitoring, it is highly likely that this monitoring approach will result in frequent false-negative findings. In essence, if syncope does not occur, but certain arrhythmias are detected (e.g., premature ventricular contractions (PVCs) or paroxysmal atrial fibrillation) the physician may be tempted to assume, incorrectly, a diagnostic connection.

Holter monitoring may be of more value in the syncope evaluation if symptoms are very frequent. Single or multiple episodes of loss of consciousness occurring on a daily basis might increase the potential for symptom–ECG correlation. However, experience in these patients (i.e., those with multiple daily events) suggests that it is unlikely that they have true syncope; indeed many of these patients may have psychogenic "black-outs" (i.e., psychogenic "pseudo-syncope"). On the other hand, in such patients, true negative (i.e., not an arrhythmic origin) findings during Holter monitoring may be useful in ruling out a cardiovascular collapse, and suggesting a psychogenic underlying cause.

External AECG event monitoring

True syncope tends to recur with a frequency of weeks or months (or even less often). Most syncope patients experience relatively long asymptomatic periods between events. Consequently, external AECG recorders that are available to the patient over these relatively long time periods would be expected to have a higher diagnostic yield than does a 24- or 48-h recording obtainable with a Holter monitor. These latter AECG recorders are commonly termed "event recorders" as they are available (in theory) for the patient to use when a symptom "event" occurs.

Conventional "event" recorders are external devices equipped with fixed electrodes through which an ECG can be recorded by direct application of the recorder electrodes to the chest wall (or other locations such as the wrist). Provided the patient can comply at the time of symptoms, a high-fidelity recording can be made.

Recordings can be prospective or retrospective or both. Some recorders have long-term cutaneous ECG patch connections, facilitating good skin contact for recordings. Newer devices can record every beat over 7 days, allowing automatic recording supplemented by patient event notification for longer periods. Often, however, patients consider devices that require long-term cutaneous electrodes to be a substantial inconvenience, and they are simply not tolerated. The need for the patient to remove and replace skin electrodes daily (to avoid skin damage) has considerable adverse impact on patient compliance.

External event recorders often have a limited value in syncope because the patient must be able to apply the recorder to the chest during the period of unconsciousness and activate recording. In the absence of a very prolonged premonitory warning period, or the presence of a very astute bystander, such application is impossible. Inevitably, with long-term external AECG monitoring, if there are no events over quite a long period of time, patient compliance drops. In such circumstances, the patient forgets to carry the instrument, and the recorder is then not nearby when an event does occur.

Implantable AECG event monitoring (ILRs)

Implantable loop recorders (ILRs) have been available since 1998 (Medtronic Reveal® and RevealPlus® ECG event monitors) (Fig. 8.1). These devices are placed in a small subcutaneous pocket analogous to the technique for placement of a conventional pacemaker generator, but without the need for vascular access as there are no leads. The optimal location is usually just to the left of the sternum. The best orientation can be "mapped" out preoperatively. The procedure is undertaken using local anesthetic, and the patient can return home almost immediately thereafter. The battery life is approximately 18–24 months.

High-fidelity ILR ECG recordings can be obtained in most patients with relatively little interference from skeletal muscle artifact or extraneous electrical "noise". The ILR has a solid state loop memory, and the current version can store up to 42 min of continuous ECG. Retrospective ECG allows activation of the device after consciousness has been restored, and the RevealPlus® version is capable of both automatic recordings (based on

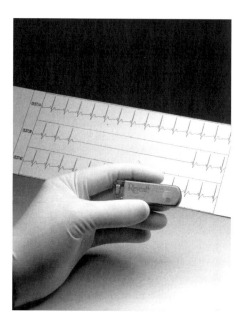

Fig. 8.1 Photograph depicting a Reveal® implantable loop recorder (Medtronic Inc., Minneapolis, MN). The small size can be inferred from the fingers holding the device.

physician-determined recording parameters) and patient-activated record-ings. In one series of very symptomatic patients, symptom–ECG correlation was achieved in approx-imately 90% of patients within 6 months of implanta-tion. Other studies of ILR use in syncope patients have resulted in a diagnostic yield of 25–40% over a 8–10-month recording period. Obviously, the more prolonged the monitoring time, the greater the chance of obtaining a useful recording.

The advantages of the ILR include continuous high-fidelity ECG recording (Figs 8.2 & 8.3), and a loop memory. The loop memory allows the patient to activate the device after consciousness is restored, and thereby retain the critical ECG recording obtained during symptoms. Further, the ILR eliminates certain logistical factors which prevent good ECG recording during symptoms, e.g., poor skin contact. The result is a high yield in terms of symptom–ECG correlation. This is because of the very long duration of monitoring (battery life 18–24 months) which confers a high likelihood of recording dur-ing recurrence of presenting symptoms. Limitations of current ILRs include the need for surgical implantation, a lack of recording of any other concurrent physiologic parameter, e.g., blood pressure, and the relatively high up-front cost of the device (Table 8.1).

Crude analysis suggests that the implantable loop recorder carries a high up-front cost. However, if symptom–ECG correlation can be achieved in 90% of patients within 6 months of implantation, then analysis of the cost per symptom–ECG yield would show that the implanted device is more cost-effective than Holter monitoring. In this regard, we analyzed costs in

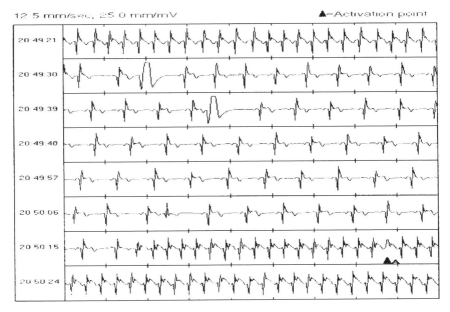

Fig. 8.2 ECG recording derived from an ILR in a syncope patient revealing that a supraventricular tachycardia was the cause of symptoms.

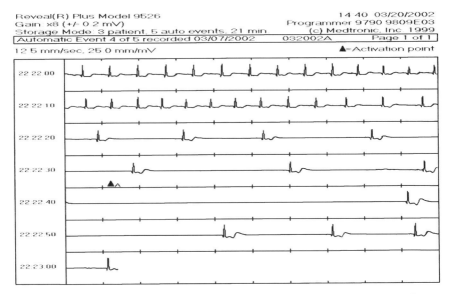

Fig. 8.3 ILR ECG tracing from a syncope patient revealing symptomatic bradycardia.

Table 8.1 Advantages and limitations of current generation implantable loop recorders.

Advantages

Prolonged ECG recording capability (18–24 months)

Loop memory—allows activation after consciousness is restored

Automatic recording—allows automatic acquisition of ECG events which fall outside programmable boundaries

Elimination of technical factors which impair good-quality surface ECG recording during symptoms (e.g., poor contact, incapacitated patient)

High symptom–ECG correlation yield (cost-effective)—prolonged recording duration increases likelihood of capturing a spontaneous event

Limitations

Need to implant the device surgically

Up-front cost—although proven "cost-effective" because of improved diagnostic yield

Lack of recording of other potentially important physiologic parameters (e.g., blood pressure)

Absence of treatment capability or long-distance communication* should a life-threatening rhythm be detected.

* Systems are currently in development that will address this limitation.

200 patients with recurrent syncope. The yield of conventional Holter ECG monitoring was 1%, while a cohort of 186 patients had 90% symptom–ECG correlation at 6 months after ILR implantation. Overall, conventional Holter monitoring cost 3.75 times as much per symptom–ECG correlation as did the ILR. Even if the ILR yield was only 30–40% it would retain a significant cost-effectiveness advantage.

AECG monitoring in syncope—where in the work-up?

The role of AECG monitoring in and the appropriate type of monitor to select for the syncope evaluation cannot be determined in isolation. Physicians should be guided by the clinical history (i.e., frequency and severity of episodes), physical examination and objective testing, for example, by head-up tilt. For some situations where evidence is accumulated this way, and strongly suggests perhaps a neurally mediated reflex syncope, AECG monitoring may be deemed unnecessary. This might be especially the case if symptoms are infrequent (i.e., Holter monitoring is particularly unlikely to yield a diagnosis), and there is a bias against implantable monitoring (e.g., young patient, patient adverse to procedures, economic issues in the health care system). In other circumstances, where treatment decisions cannot be made without more information, recording a spontaneous event becomes crucial. In the future, as technology allows recording of multiple signals in addition to the

ECG, greater emphasis will be placed on the features of spontaneous, rather than provoked (i.e., tilt-table or electrophysiologic study (EPS)), syncope.

ILRs will likely become increasingly important in the evaluation of syncope patients. Knowing what transpires during a spontaneous syncopal episode is the gold standard for the syncope evaluation. In some instances, the ILR has taught us definitively the cause of syncope, such that any further investigation has become redundant. However, the current ILR represents only a first step. Documentation of blood pressure as well as other physiologic measures (see later) may offer additional insight into syncope mechanisms.

Recommendations

Often the cause(s) of syncope can be identified by application of careful medical history-taking and routine low-cost investigations (e.g., resting 12-lead ECG and echocardiography). However, with these tools alone, there remains a high rate of "unknowns". AECG monitoring, when used prudently, can be very effective in increasing the diagnostic yield. However, the choice of monitoring strategy requires some thought.

Patients with very infrequent syncope, recurring over months or years, are unlikely to be diagnosed by conventional Holter monitoring, since the likelihood of symptom–ECG correlation during a 24–48-h recording period is very low. Consideration should be given to conventional event recording in such patients. However, it has to be acknowledged that conventional external recorders have important logistical limitations (such as being able to activate the device) that diminish their effectiveness during syncope. In such circumstances, and especially those cases in which the interval between recurrences is measured in months or years, consideration must be given to implanting an AECG loop recorder (ILR). The vast majority of ILR patients provide symptom–ECG correlation within a year of device placement. Consequently, despite the up-front device cost, ILRs have proved to be cost-effective on a diagnostic yield basis when compared to Holter monitoring or even conventional external event monitoring.

Summary

The most potent investigation in a syncope patient is the one that records a clear abnormality at the time when the presenting symptoms are reproduced. It is important to strive to achieve this with AECG monitoring. Expanded ILR use appears to be the most important step forward in this regard. Where symptoms are not reproduced but an ECG abnormality is found, there will always be doubt about the true diagnosis. Nevertheless, sometimes it is necessary to act on the basis of an asymptomatic finding. Future refinements to technology, such as the ability to record systemic pressure and patient posture and activity status, may help remove such doubts.

Further reading

Crawford MH, Bernstein SJ, Deedwania PC *et al*. ACC/AHA guidelines for ambulatory electrocardiography. *J Am Coll Cardiol* 1999; 34: 912–948. (Executive summary and recommendations. *Circulation* 1999; 100: 886–893.)

Krahn AD, Klein GJ, Yee R, Takle-Newhouse T, Norris C. Use of an extended monitoring strategy in patients with problematic syncope. Reveal Investigators. *Circulation* 1999; 26: 99: 406–410.

Seidl K, Ramekan M, Breuning S *et al*. Diagnostic assessment of recurrent unexplained syncope with a new subcutaneously implantable loop recorder. *Europace* 2000; 2: 256–262.

Moya A, Brignole M, Menozzi C *et al*. Mechanism of syncope in patients with isolated syncope and in patients with tilt-positive syncope. *Circulation* 2001; 104: 1261–1267.

Krahn A, Klein GJ, Yee R, Skanes AC. Randomized assessment of syncope trial. Conventional diagnostic testing versus a prolonged monitoring strategy. *Circulation* 2001; 104: 46–51.

CHAPTER 9

The basic autonomic assessment

Richard Sutton, David G Benditt

Introduction

The neurally mediated syncopal syndromes are the most frequent of all causes of syncope. Since these conditions reflect a transient functional change in autonomic system function, it is reasonable to utilize tools designed to assess such function as part of the diagnostic assessment in syncope patients.

A detailed discussion of the various neurally mediated syncope syndromes is provided elsewhere in this volume (see Chapters 1, 2 & 14, Part 1). However, with respect to identifying susceptibility to the most important of these (i.e., vasovagal syncope and carotid sinus syndrome), certain tests are now well established and widely available. The most important of these tests are: (i) head-up tilt testing; and (ii) carotid sinus massage. Less well delineated in terms of utility are: (i) Valsalva maneuver; (ii) active standing test; (iii) cold pressor test; (iv) eyeball compression test; (v) response to cough; (vi) heart rate variability assessment; and (vii) ATP/adenosine test. The last two of these tests are discussed in Chapter 11, and will not be considered here.

Goals

The goals of this chapter are to provide a review of the technique, utility and limitations of:
- head-up tilt-table testing;
- carotid sinus massage;
- Valsalva maneuver;
- active standing test; and
- cough test.

Vasovagal syncope and head-up tilt-table testing

Vasovagal syncope may be triggered by any of a variety of factors (see Chapter 14, Part 1). Some of the latter include unpleasant sights (e.g., sight of blood),

Table 9.1 Recommended tilt test protocols.

Supine pretilt phase of 10 min when no venous cannulation is performed, and at least 20 min when cannulation is undertaken

A passive phase of minimum of 20 min and a maximum of 45 min followed by a drug challenge phase, if necessary, of 15–20 min is recommended

The recommended tilt angle is 60–70 degrees

Either intravenous isoproterenol or sublingual nitroglycerin is recommended for drug provocation

The recommended infusion rate for isoproterenol is incremental doses from 1 up to 3 µg/min in order to increase average heart rate by about 20–25% over baseline, administered without returning the patient to a supine position

The recommended dose for nitroglycerin challenge is 400 µg nitroglycerin spray sublingually

A positive end-point of the test is defined as induction of syncope, or reproduction of symptoms in association with near-syncope symptoms

---

pain, extreme emotion, prolonged standing, stuffy rooms, boredom, and the previous consumption of alcohol. Typical venues for fainting are churches, hospitals, the sports field (usually in association with injury), parties, queues (i.e., standing in line for prolonged period of time), traveling by air, and restaurants.

Vasovagal syncope is often suspected as a result of the clinical history; however, this is not always possible. Consequently, the availability of a test assessing susceptibility to vasovagal syncope, namely the head-up tilt-table test, is of value (Table 9.1).

Detailed discussion of tilt-table testing protocols, test reproducibility, and estimated specificity and sensitivity, are best found in the ACC Expert Consensus Report and the recent guidelines document from the European Society of Cardiology (see "Further reading" section below). As a rule, the first step is "passive" head-up tilt at 60–70 degrees during which the patient is supported by a foot-plate and gently applied body straps for a period of not less than 20 and perhaps as long as 45 min. Tilt angles of less than 60 and greater than 80 degrees lead to loss of sensitivity and specificity. Subsequently, if needed, tilt testing in conjunction with a drug challenge (e.g., isoproterenol, edrophonium, nitroglycerin) may be undertaken either immediately or as a separate procedure. This is particularly pertinent if a short passive phase is used (i.e., 20–30 min). Until recently, the most frequently used provocative drug was isoproterenol usually given in escalating doses from 1 to 3 µg/min. However, nitroglycerin intravenously or sublingually has gained favor, in part because it expedites the procedure without adversely affecting diagnostic utility. Additionally, sublingual nitroglycerin can be administered without a parenteral canula.

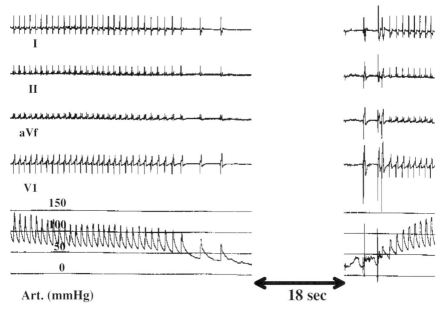

I

II

aVf

V1

150

100

50

0

Art. (mmHg)   **18 sec**

Fig. 9.1 ECG and blood pressure recordings during a tilt-table-induced vasovagal faint. Note gradual drop in blood pressure prior to development of a long asystolic pause. Several seconds of asystole have been removed from the recording. Return of the patient to supine posture (right side of tracing) results in prompt termination of the event and restoration of normal hemodynamics.

The head-up tilt-table test is the only readily available test which provides the opportunity to precipitate a typical vasovagal attack under the eyes of the physician (Fig. 9.1). As a result, it helps the patient by giving confidence that the physician has witnessed the problem, and it also provides the patient with valuable experience which may help recognition of impending faints and thereby avert future events. Nonetheless, tilt-table testing is imperfect. The false-positive rate is approximately 10%. Acute (i.e., same day or within a few days) test reproducibility in terms of whether syncope is induced or not is approximately 80–90%. Longer-term reproducibility (i.e., over more than 1 year) is around 60%. Since there is no "gold standard" for diagnosis of neurally mediated syncope, the sensitivity of tilt testing cannot accurately be estimated.

It has been known for some time that tilt testing does not always result in the same hemodynamic picture when repeated in the same patient (Table 9.2). Thus, cardioinhibition (i.e., bradycardia) may predominate on one occasion whereas vasodilatation with hypotension may occur at another time. Thus, tilt testing may not be optimal for directing treatment strategy. In this regard, the recently published ISSUE study indicates that even when tilt testing showed a prominent vasodilatory component to the faint, the subsequent recording

Table 9.2 Classifications of positive responses to tilt testing (based on VASIS group).

Type 1 Mixed. Heart rate falls at the time of syncope but the ventricular rate does not fall to less than 40 beats/min or falls to less than 40 beats/min for less than 10 sec with or without asystole of less than 3 sec. Blood pressure falls before the heart rate falls

Type 2A Cardioinhibition without asystole. Heart rate falls to a ventricular rate less than 40 beats/min for more than 10 sec but asystole of more than 3 sec does not occur. Blood pressure falls before the heart rate falls

Type 2B Cardioinhibition with asystole. Asystole occurs for more than 3 sec. Blood pressure fall coincides with or occurs before the heart rate fall

Type 3 Vasodepressor. Heart rate does not fall more than 10% from its peak at the time of syncope

Exception 1. Chronotropic incompetence. No heart rate rise during the tilt testing (i.e., less than 10% from the pretilt rate)

Exception 2. Excessive heart rate rise. An excessive heart rate rise both at the onset of upright position and throughout its duration before syncope (i.e., greater than 130 beats/min)

of spontaneous faints by means of an implantable loop recorder (ILR) often revealed bradycardic events. Further study of this phenomenon with devices which can monitor blood pressure (or a surrogate of blood pressure), as well as heart rate is needed.

Independent of the protocol employed, certain general measures can be suggested when tilt testing is performed:

- The room where the test is performed should be quiet and with dim lights.
- Patients should fast for at least 2 h before the test.
- Patients should be in a supine position 10–45 min before tilting. This longer time interval was proposed to decrease the likelihood of a vasovagal reaction in response to venous cannulation. The shorter rest periods (e.g., 10 min) are proposed when vascular cannulation is not employed.
- Continuous beat-to-beat finger arterial blood pressure should be monitored non-invasively, if reliable recordings can be obtained. Intermittent measurement of pressure using a sphygmomanometer should be avoided as it is disruptive to the procedure, and the frequency of recording is too low. Nevertheless, the latter method is used in clinical practice, especially in children.
- The tilt-table should be able to achieve the upright position smoothly and rapidly and to reset to the supine position quickly (< 10 sec) when the test is completed in order to avoid the consequences of a prolonged loss of consciousness. Only a tilt-table of the foot-board support type is appropriate for syncope evaluation.
- An experienced nurse or medical technician should be in attendance during the entire procedure. A physician should be in proximity and immediately

available should a problem arise. Resuscitation equipment should be immediately available.

Role of head-up tilt test in treatment selection for vasovagal syncope

In order for any test to be helpful in the evaluation of treatment, the test must exhibit a high degree of reproducibility and be predictive of outcomes at follow-up. The overall reproducibility of an initial negative response (85–94%) is higher than the reproducibility of an initial positive response (31–92%). In addition, data from controlled trials showed that approximately 50% of patients with a baseline positive tilt test became negative when the test was repeated with treatment or with placebo. Moreover, in most cases acute studies were not predictive of the long-term outcome of pacing therapy. Thus, it is generally agreed that head-up tilt testing is best reserved for diagnostic testing and is not considered to be of value for assessment of treatment options.

Complications

Head-up tilt test is a safe procedure and the rate of complications is very low. Although asystolic pauses > 70 sec have been reported, the presence of such prolonged asystole during a positive response cannot be considered a complication, since this is an end-point of the test. Rapid return to supine position as soon as syncope occurs is usually all that is needed to prevent or to limit the consequences of prolonged loss of consciousness. Only seldom are brief resuscitation maneuvers required. The mortality rate associated with tilt-table testing is not known. However, reports of deaths are exceedingly rare, and the mortality rate is likely < 1/100,000 tests.

Case reports have documented life-threatening ventricular arrhythmias with isoproterenol in the presence of ischemic heart disease or sick sinus syndrome. No complications have been published with the use of nitroglycerin.

Indications

Tilt testing is indicated for diagnostic purposes. It is not recommended for assessments of treatment efficacy.

Indications for tilt testing include:
- unexplained recurrent or single syncopal episode in the absence of organic heart disease in high-risk clinical settings (see text for discussion);
- unexplained recurrent or single syncopal episode in the presence of organic heart disease, after cardiac causes of syncope have been excluded;
- after an etiology of syncope has been established, but where the demonstration of susceptibility to neurally mediated syncope would alter the therapeutic approach.

Tilt testing may be useful for:
- differentiating syncope with jerking movements from epilepsy;
- evaluating patients with recurrent unexplained falls;
- assessing recurrent presyncope or dizziness;

- evaluating unexplained syncope in the setting of peripheral neuropathies or autonomic failure; and
- postexercise-related syncope when an attack cannot be documented by exercise testing.

For patients without severe structural heart disease, tilt testing can be considered diagnostic, and no further tests need to be performed, when spontaneous syncope is reproduced. For patients with significant structural heart disease, arrhythmias should be excluded as a cause prior to considering positive tilt test results as evidence suggesting neurally mediated syncope. The clinical meaning of abnormal responses other than induction of syncope is unclear.

Carotid sinus syndrome and carotid sinus massage

Carotid sinus syndrome usually presents with syncope without warning. Although rare, a history suggesting that head movements trigger dizziness or syncope supports this diagnosis. As a rule, the condition almost exclusively afflicts older people with substantial male dominance. This is in contrast to vasovagal syncope; the latter tends to affect the sexes equally and occurs at all ages.

It has long been known that pressure at the site where the common carotid artery bifurcates produces a reflex slowing in heart rate and fall in blood pressure. This observation is the basis of the technique of carotid sinus massage (CSM). In some patients with syncope, an exaggerated response to CSM can be observed. In the absence of a history of spontaneous syncope, the exaggerated response is defined as carotid sinus hypersensitivity, and must be distinguished from carotid sinus syndrome.

Methodology and response to carotid sinus massage

CSM is typically performed initially with the patient in a supine position. However, it is recommended that both supine and upright positions (usually on a tilt-table) be tested. Continuous ECG monitoring must be used. Continuous blood pressure monitoring is also desirable as the vasodepressor response is rapid and cannot be adequately detected with devices which do not measure continuous blood pressure. For the latter measurement, a non-invasive device is often suitable but conventional blood pressure cuff recordings are not.

After baseline measurements, the right carotid artery is firmly massaged for 5–10 sec at the anterior margin of the sternocleidomastoid muscle at the level of the cricoid cartilage. After 1 or 2 min a second massage is performed on the opposite side if the massage on one side failed to yield a "positive" result. If an asystolic response is evoked, it may be helpful to repeat the massage after intravenous administration of atropine (1 mg or 0.02 mg/kg) in order to assess the contribution of the vasodepressor component (which may otherwise be hidden). Atropine administration is preferred to temporary dual chamber pacing as it is simple, less invasive and easily reproducible. The response to CSM is generally classified as cardioinhibitory (i.e., asystole), vasodepressive (fall in systolic blood pressure), or mixed. This latter response is more difficult to interpret and usually diagnosed as the association of an asystole of 3 sec and a decline in systolic blood pressure of 50 mmHg or more from the baseline value.

Two approaches to the diagnostic use of CSM have been advocated.

• *Method 1*: This is probably the most widely used technique in clinical practice. CSM is performed with the patient supine. Pressure is applied for no more than 5 sec. A positive response is defined as a ventricular pause ≥ 3 sec and/or a fall of systolic blood pressure ≥ 50 mmHg. Pooled data from four studies performed in elderly patients with syncope show a rate of 35% (235 of 663 patients). Abnormal responses can also be frequently observed in subjects without syncope. The diagnosis may be missed in about one third of cases if only supine massage is performed.

• *Method 2*: Reproduction of spontaneous symptoms is required during carotid massage. Eliciting symptoms requires a longer period of massage (10 sec) performed in both supine and upright positions. A positive response was observed in 49% of 100 patients with syncope of uncertain origin and in 60% of elderly patients with syncope and sinus bradycardia, but only in 4% of 101 control patients without syncope pooled from three studies.

Whatever method is used, increasing importance is now given to undertaking CSM with the patient in upright position, usually using a tilt-table. Apart from the higher positive diagnosis rate, compared to supine massage only, upright CSM better evaluates the magnitude of the vasodepressor component of the reflex; this component has been underestimated in the past, and its magnitude may affect the utility of cardiac pacing therapy.

Complications of CSM

The main complications of carotid sinus massage are neurologic. In one study, 7 neurologic complications were reported among 5000 carotid massages, with an incidence of 0.14%. In another study, 16 neurologic complications were reported in 16,000 massages (0.01%). These complication rates apply to 5 sec of CSM supine and/or upright.

CSM should be avoided in patients with previous transient ischemic attacks or strokes within the past 3 months (unless carotid Doppler studies convincingly exclude significant carotid artery narrowing), or in patients with carotid bruits. On rare occasion CSM may elicit self-limited atrial fibrillation of little clinical significance.

CSM indications

Carotid sinus massage should be performed in every patient less than 40 years of age with syncope in whom the initial evaluation is negative, and in whom there is no evident contraindication.

• CSM is recommended in patients over the age of 40 years with syncope of unknown etiology after the initial evaluation. In the case of risk of stroke due to carotid artery disease, the massage should be avoided.

- ECG monitoring and blood pressure measurement during carotid massage is mandatory. Massage should be of 5–10 sec duration. Carotid massage should be performed with the patient both supine and upright.
- A positive outcome to CSM is reported if syncope is reproduced during or immediately after the massage in the presence of asystole longer than 3 sec and/or a fall in systolic blood pressure of 50 mmHg or more.

Miscellaneous autonomic system tests

Several studies are occasionally used in the laboratory but their clinical value is as yet unclear.

Valsalva maneuver

This test is well known in medicine. Its utility lies in assessment of the integrity of certain vascular reflex responses to induced hemodynamic stress. In this sense it provides an estimate of autonomic nervous system integrity. However, Valsalva maneuver does not directly implicate a mechanism for syncope.

Active standing test

This procedure, as its name implies, assesses patient response to active movement from supine to upright posture. It may be more useful in evaluating symptoms of orthostatic intolerance than is passive head-up tilt. Normally, active muscle movement is expected to propel more blood toward the central circulation, thereby aiding the needed increase in cardiac output. However, active use of lower limb muscles may play a role in aggravating peripheral vascular dilatation and as a result induce greater hypotension. The balance between these physiologic effects of active muscle movement determines the net effect with regard to systemic pressure.

Cold pressor test

Like the Valsalva maneuver, this test provides insight into autonomic reflex integrity. It has not been used as a means of identifying a specific diagnosis.

Eyeball compression test

This test, previously used to induce a vagal reflex, should be abandoned. Its utility is low, and its clinical diagnostic benefit is marginal compared to potential risks.

Cough test

The use of induced cough to assess susceptibility to cough (tussive) syncope has been discussed, but little data is available. Like carotid massage, it may be best undertaken with the patient in the upright posture.

Summary

Well established clinical tests are available for evaluation of the role autonomic dysfunction may play as a contributing factor in syncope. For the most part, however, only head-up tilt and carotid sinus massage are of known clinical value. These tests are easily performed and have well defined end-points. They are recommended for diagnosis only, but are of more limited value for defining treatment options. The remaining tests discussed above may be helpful from time to time, but are not adequately substantiated to advocate their routine use.

Further reading

Brignole M, Alboni P, Benditt DG *et al.* Guidelines on management (diagnosis and treatment) of syncope. *Eur Heart J* 2001; 22: 1256–1306.

Sutton R, Petersen M, Brignole M *et al.* Proposed classification for tilt induced vasovagal syncope. *Eur J Cardiac Pacing Electrophysiol* 1992; 2: 180–183.

Brignole M, Menozzi C, Del Rosso A *et al.* New classification of hemodynamics of vasovagal syncope: beyond the VASIS classification. Analysis of the presyncopal phase of the tilt test without and with nitroglycerin challenge. Vasovagal Syncope International Study. *Europace* 2000; 2: 66–76.

Moya A, Brignole M, Menozzi C, Garcia-Civera R, Tognarini S, Mont L, Botto G, Giada F, Cornacchia D, and ISSUE Investigators. Mechanism of syncope in patients with isolated syncope and in patients with tilt-positive syncope. *Circulation* 2001; 104: 1261–1267.

Benditt DG, Ferguson DW, Grubb BP *et al.* Tilt-table testing for assessing syncope. An American College of Cardiology expert consensus document. *J Am Coll Cardiol* 1996; 28(1): 263–275.

Almquist A, Gornick CC, Benson DW Jr *et al.* Carotid sinus hypersensitivity: evaluation of the vasodepressor component. *Circulation* 1985; 67: 927–936.

CHAPTER 10

Role of electrophysiologic testing in the syncope evaluation

Fei Lu, Lennart Bergfeldt

Introduction

The role of invasive electrophysiologic study (EPS) in the evaluation of the syncope patient is primarily to confirm a clinical suspicion (derived from the initial evaluation) that a primary cardiac rhythm abnormality or conduction disturbance is the likely cause of syncope in a given individual. This is accomplished by demonstrating that an arrhythmia substrate or clinically significant conduction disturbance is present, and in the absence of other explanation, inferring a relationship between the abnormality and syncope. On occasion, EPS techniques (especially mapping and ablation) may also play an important role in treatment and prevention.

Goals

The goals of this chapter are to:
- review briefly the most important EPS techniques;
- discuss the diagnostic utility and limitations of EPS; and
- examine a number of specific clinical conditions associated with syncope in which EPS may be of value.

Methodology

With regard to the role of cardiac arrhythmias as a cause of syncope, both bradycardias (sinus node dysfunction and/or atrioventricular (AV) block) and tachycardias (ventricular or supraventricular) can be at fault. EPS may be helpful in focusing on the most likely arrhythmic cause, and directing choices for treatment. However, in the absence of clinical suspicion, EPS is not a reliable screening tool. This is particularly true for patients without structural heart disease.

For the most part, EPS requires placement of one or more electrode catheters into the heart using conventional vascular access techniques. Most studies require only venous access (usually the femoral vein) to record from and electrically stimulate the right atrium, right ventricle and occasionally the coronary sinus vein which wraps around the left atrium. However, arterial access with recording from and stimulation of the left ventricle is occasionally needed. Transesophageal EPS is also used from time to time, particularly in children. Since the transesophageal electrode predominantly records and stimulates on the atrial level, it is limited in its utility to screening for conditions which primarily involve atrial tissues (e.g., sinus node dysfunction, paroxysmal supraventricular tachycardias—PSVT).

One of the distinct advantages of EPS is the potential to identify and cure certain arrhythmias during the same session. In this regard, transcatheter ablation using radiofrequency energy is now an integral part of the capabilities of most EPS laboratories, and can be used to cure several arrhythmias that may cause syncope (* indicates rarely a cause of syncope), such as:

- rapid heart rhythms associated with Wolff–Parkinson–White syndrome (WPW syndrome) or other forms of ventricular pre-excitation or accessory pathway-mediated tachycardia (including so-called "Mahaim" nodoventricular and nodofascicular connections*, and the permanent form of junctional reciprocating tachycardia—PJRT*);
- PSVT due to AV node re-entry;
- certain primary ectopic atrial tachycardias*, and to a lesser extent inappropriate sinus tachycardia* and sinoatrial re-entry*;
- atrial flutter, and some cases of atrial fibrillation*; and
- several forms of idiopathic ventricular tachycardia arising from the right or left ventricles:
  bundle branch re-entry tachycardia
  right ventricular outflow tract (and more rarely left ventricular outflow tract) tachycardia (see also Chapter 14, Part 3) and
  fascicular tachycardias.

For patients with unexplained syncope, following evaluation of baseline clinical history and non-invasive testing, EPS is commonly used to assess susceptibility to a priori suspected sinus node function, AV conduction disturbances and/or various tachyarrhythmias. As a rule, in patients with a normal resting electrocardiogram (ECG), no evident structural heart disease, and a history of syncope associated with palpitations, EPS is best for assessing susceptibility to PSVT as the probable cause of syncope. On the other hand, for patients with an abnormal ECG and/or evidence of structural heart disease, cardiac conduction system disease and ventricular arrhythmias are a greater concern.

In all patients, neurally mediated reflex syncope (in all its forms, see Chapter 14, Part 1) and orthostatic syncope (see Chapter 14, Part 2) need to be carefully considered as possible causes of syncope since they are so common. This is particularly the case in older patients in whom more than one cause may exist. However, these conditions are not appropriate for evaluation by

Table 10.1 Guideline recommendations for electrophysiologic testing indications.

Class I
An invasive EPS procedure is indicated when the initial evaluation suggests an arrhythmic cause of syncope. Risk factors include abnormal electrocardiography, structural heart disease, syncope associated with palpitations, and family history of sudden death.

Class II
Diagnostic reasons: to evaluate the exact nature (mechanisms) of an arrhythmia which has already been identified as the cause of the syncope.
Prognostic reasons:
1 In patients with cardiac disease, in which arrhythmia induction has a bearing on the selection of therapy.
2 In patients with high-risk occupations, in whom every effort to exclude a cardiac cause of syncope is warranted.

Class III
In patients without abnormal electrocardiograms, structural heart disease or palpitations, EPS is not usually indicated.

Note:
1 Normal EPS findings cannot completely exclude an arrhythmic cause of syncope. When an arrhythmia is still suspected after a negative EPS, further evaluations (such as loop recording) are recommended (class I).
2 Abnormal electrocardiographic findings may not be diagnostic of the cause of syncope depending on the clinical context.

Table 10.2 Minimal suggested electrophysiologic protocol for diagnosis of syncope.

Measurement of sinus node recovery time and corrected sinus node recovery time by repeated sequences of atrial pacing for 30–60 sec with at least one low and two high pacing rates. Suggested low pacing rate is 10–20 beats above sinus rate. Autonomic blockade may be applied if needed (see text for doses).

Assessment of the His–Purkinje system includes measurement of the HV at baseline and His–Purkinje conduction with stress by incremental atrial pacing. If HV interval is moderately prolonged, pharmacologic provocation is recommended unless contraindicated. Suggested drugs include ajmaline 1 mg/kg or procainamide 10 mg/kg.

Assessment of ventricular arrhythmia inducibility performed by programmed electrical stimulation using up to two extrastimuli (with coupling interval not below 200 ms) from two right ventricular sites (apex and outflow tract) at two drive cycle lengths (100 or 120 beats/min and 140 or 150 beats/min). A third extrastimulus may be added to enhance sensitivity at the cost of reduced specificity.

Assessment of supraventricular arrhythmia inducibility by any atrial stimulation protocols.

conventional EPS. Autonomic testing and head-up tilt testing are required (see Chapter 9 & Chapter 14, Parts 1 & 2). These latter tests, along with the appropriate evaluation of other possible causes of syncope, are considered in other chapters in this book. Indications for EPS in the evaluation of syncope patients are summarized in Table 10.1, and the minimum procedure requirements are provided in Table 10.2.

Diagnostic yield and predictive value

The gold standard for the diagnosis of arrhythmia-related syncope is ECG documentation of episodes of spontaneous cardiac arrhythmias causing syncope. However, in many patients with unexplained syncope, EPS is able to elicit a possible diagnosis of a suspected cardiac arrhythmia. This is particularly the case in those individuals with an abnormal ECG and/or evident underlying structural heart disease. Nevertheless, in the absence of reproduction of symptoms, the observations must remain only a presumptive cause of syncope.

The diagnostic efficiency of EPS is highly dependent on the degree of suspicion of the abnormality (pretest probability), the aggressiveness of the protocol, and the criteria used for diagnosis of clinically significant abnormalities. The diagnostic yield of EPS has not been fully evaluated by assessing concordance with diagnoses determined by other techniques such as ambulatory ECG monitoring (Chapter 8). Table 10.3 provides a list of findings during EPS that are highly likely to suggest a correct diagnosis in a syncope patient.

Table 10.3 Diagnostic findings during EPS.

EPS is diagnostic and usually no additional tests are needed
1 Significant sinus bradycardia and a markedly prolonged corrected sinus node recovery time (> 800 ms).
2 Bifascicular block associated with one of the following:
   (i) A baseline HV interval of 100 ms, or greater.
  (ii) 2nd or 3rd degree His–Purkinje block is demonstrated during incremental atrial pacing at moderate heart rates.
 (iii) High-degree His–Purkinje block is provoked by pharmacologic challenge.
 (iv) Induction of monomorphic ventricular tachycardia in patients with prior myocardial infarction.
  (v) Induction of ventricular tachycardia/ventricular fibrillation in patients with arrhythmogenic right ventricular dysplasia.
 (vi) Induction of rapid supraventricular tachycardias with hypotensive responses and clinical symptoms.

Divergence of opinion exists on the diagnostic value of EPS in the following settings
1 HV interval is moderately prolonged (70–100 ms).
2 Induction of polymorphic ventricular tachycardia and ventricular fibrillation in both ischemic and non-ischemic dilated cardiomyopathies.
3 In Brugada syndrome.

EPS limitations

EPS is most effective for delineating fixed cardiac conduction defects (e.g., AV block due to His–Purkinje system disease), and susceptibility to re-entrant tachycardias (e.g., PSVT, many forms of ventricular tachycardia). However, EPS sensitivity with conservative criteria (sinus node recovery time > 3000 ms) in identifying transient rhythm disturbances, especially bradycardias, is low (15%) in syncope patients. Furthermore, abnormal sinus and AV node function unrelated to syncope may be found and unrelated supraventricular or ventricular tachyarrhythmias may be induced in many of these patients. These findings may be mistaken as the cause of syncope. However, if neurally mediated reflex syncope and orthostatic syncope have been excluded, then evidence of susceptibility to significant bradycardia (i.e., abnormal sinus node or His–Purkinje function) appears to provide a reasonable diagnosis in the majority of patients (86%) with spontaneous syncope due to sinus arrest or paroxysmal AV block. Recent studies using electrocardiographic monitoring before EPS or monitoring function of a pacemaker after EPS support this observation.

As noted earlier, EPS tends to be most helpful in patients with known structural heart disease. Thus, ventricular tachycardia was induced in 21% and abnormal indices of bradycardia were found in 34% of patients with organic heart disease or an abnormal standard ECG. In contrast, abnormal electrophysiologic findings are much lower (ventricular tachycardia 1% and bradycardia 10%) in patients with an apparently normal heart. Nevertheless, in all cases, the physician must carefully consider whether the EPS findings are consistent with the clinical history, or whether they may be a false positive. In general, EPS has been less effective in identifying bradycardic causes of syncope than tachycardic causes.

Specific clinical conditions

Suspected sinus node dysfunction

A transient symptomatic bradycardia due to sinus node dysfunction (also termed sick sinus syndrome, and sinus node disease) should be suspected in evaluating a patient with syncope when there is an asymptomatic sinus bradycardia (< 50 beats/min) or sinoatrial "pauses" (usually considered abnormal if > 3 sec duration), or a prolonged asystole after spontaneous termination or cardioversion of atrial fibrillation (Fig. 10.1). However, although these findings may be very suspicious, in the absence of occurrence of symptoms at the time of the documented arrhythmia, they can only be considered as inferential in terms of the cause of syncope (Fig. 10.2).

EPS assessment of sinus node function should include assessment of sinus automaticity (heart rate, sinus node recovery time, intrinsic heart rate). Other available but clinically less effective measures of sinus node function include sinoatrial conduction time, and sinus node refractoriness. Assessment of sinus

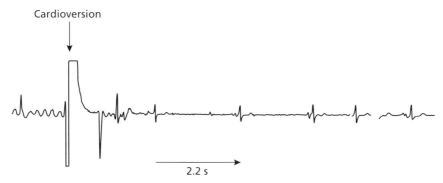

Fig. 10.1 ECG recording obtained during elective cardioversion of atrial fibrillation/flutter. After the cardioversion shock there is a brief period of disorganized atrial rhythm followed by termination of atrial fibrillation. A several-second pause follows (note blocked P wave) after which there are several junctional (short "PR" interval) beats prior to emergence of a true sinus beat (note the deformed P wave). This patient had symptomatic bradycardia–tachycardia form of sinus node dysfunction.

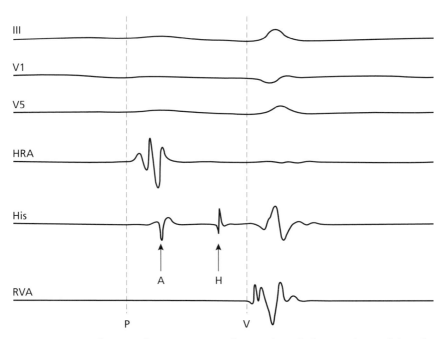

Fig. 10.2 ECG and intracardiac tracings revealing a relatively long HV interval (i.e., the conduction time from the His bundle to the ventricles). This suggests the presence of conduction system disease.

node refractoriness is not yet clinically useful. Sinoatrial conduction time is an insensitive indicator of sinus node dysfunction (prolonged in 40% of patients with clinical findings of sinus node dysfunction) and cannot always be assessed in patients with proven sinus node disease.

Sinus node recovery time is the most useful method for assessment of sinus node function. It is imperative to understand that these tests are only indirect and impure analysis of sinus node function. Sinus node recovery time is usually corrected for baseline heart rate (corrected sinus node recovery time). Sinus node recovery time > 1500–1720 ms or corrected sinus node recovery time > 525 ms is considered abnormal, with sensitivity of 50–80% and specificity of > 95%, respectively, for detecting sinus node dysfunction.

Abnormal sinus node recovery time or sinoatrial conduction time may be due to either intrinsic sinus node disease or extrinsic autonomic or drug influences. Autonomic blockade by administration of atropine and propranolol is accepted for distinguishing between intrinsic and extrinsic sinus node dysfunction. When the baseline study is inconclusive, pharmacologic interventions may increase sensitivity. Complete autonomic blockade, aimed at unmasking intrinsic sinus node function, can be achieved by administration of intravenous propranolol (0.2 mg/kg) and atropine (0.04 mg/kg). Note, however, that for the elderly the risk for adverse effects of atropine is high. In these patients, autonomic inhibition with half the conventional dose is advisable.

Intrinsic heart rate (i.e., heart rate after complete autonomic blockade) has a linear relationship to age, equal to $118.1 - (0.57 \times age)$. However, the sensitivity of abnormal intrinsic heart rate alone is low for diagnosing sinus node dysfunction. On the other hand, the use of EPS stimulation procedures (see above) for assessment of sinus node function is more reliable and reproducible after autonomic blockade.

The prognostic value of a prolonged sinus node recovery time is largely unknown. The percentage of patients with suspected sinus node dysfunction in whom sinus node recovery time has been reported to be abnormal has varied considerably in published reports. The efficacy of pacing on symptoms is associated with prolonged sinus node recovery time. Its predictive value increases with longer sinus node recovery time. Patients with a corrected sinus node recovery time of > 800 ms have an 8 times higher risk of syncope than patients with a corrected sinus node recovery time below this value. It is the opinion of the ESC Syncope Task Force panel that, in the presence of a sinus node recovery time > 2.0 sec or corrected sinus node recovery time > 1 sec, sinus node dysfunction may be reasonably surmised to be the cause of syncope if no other diagnostic candidates remain.

Suspected impending high-degree atrioventricular block

Transient high-degree AV block should be suspected in patients with syncope in the presence of bundle branch block. Extended electrocardiographic monitoring is often needed to document the transient high-degree AV block. The ISSUE study provides strong evidence of the potential importance of transient AV block as a cause of syncope in patients with bundle branch block on ECG.

The most alarming ECG sign in a patient with syncope is probably the alternating complete left and right bundle branch block, or alternating right bundle branch block with left anterior or posterior fascicular block. This ECG pattern suggests trifascicular conduction system disease and intermittent or impending high-degree AV block. Bifascicular block (right bundle branch block plus left anterior or posterior fascicular block, or left bundle branch block) is also associated with high risk of developing high-degree AV block.

EPS is used mainly to evaluate intra- and infra-His conduction (i.e., the portion of the conduction system below the AV node) in these patients (Fig. 10.1). A prolonged HV interval or a split His potential (rare) is associated with a higher risk of developing AV block. The progression rate to AV block is 2–4% in patients with normal (< 55 ms) or slightly prolonged (55–60 ms) HV intervals, and increases to 21% and 24% when the HV interval is 70 ms and 100 ms, respectively. Incremental atrial pacing and pharmacologic provocation with antiarrhythmic drugs (e.g., ajmaline, procainamide) are often used to increase the diagnostic yield of EPS when HV interval is borderline prolonged.

Development of intra- or infra-His block during incremental atrial pacing (i.e., pacing the atria at progressively more rapid rates to stress the adequacy of the AV conduction system) is highly predictive of impending AV block. Progression to complete AV block occurs in 30–40% of these patients over 2–4 years follow-up. However, its sensitivity is low (< 10%). In patients with moderate prolongation of the HV interval, pharmacologic stress testing of the His–Purkinje system may be used to assess His–Purkinje system reserve by acute intravenous administration of class Ia agents (ajmaline 1 mg/kg, procainamide 10 mg/kg). A significant increase of HV interval duration (i.e., a resultant HV > 100 ms or the precipitation of 2nd or 3rd degree intra- or infra-His block) following pharmacologic challenge with or without incremental atrial pacing is highly predictive of subsequent spontaneous AV block during follow-up. Pooled data ($n = 333$) show that pharmacologic stress was able to elicit susceptibility to high-degree AV block in 15% of patients studied. Spontaneous AV block developed in approximately 68% of these patients during follow-up for a period of 2–5 years.

With regard to the role of cardiac conduction system disease as a cause of syncope, combining the above-mentioned protocols should be able to yield a predictive value of 80% or higher. Pacemaker therapy effectively prevents recurrences of syncope in almost all these patients, indicating the value of EPS in the management of patients with syncope. A small percentage (< 20%) of the patients with negative EPS may nonetheless develop AV block during follow-up.

A high incidence of death or sudden cardiac death has been observed in patients with bundle branch block, especially in the presence of structural heart disease. Age, congestive heart failure and coronary artery disease are associated with higher risk of death. Neither syncope nor a prolonged HV interval is associated with high risk of death. Pacemaker therapy does not decrease this risk. The mechanism of sudden cardiac death is believed to be due to ventricular tachyarrhythmia or electromechanical dissociation rather than a bradycardia. A sustained ventricular tachyarrhythmia is frequently induced in patients with bundle branch block (32%).

It is the opinion of the ESC Syncope Task Force panel that, for patients with syncope and bifascicular block, EPS is highly sensitive in identifying patients with intermittent or impending high-degree AV block. This block is likely the cause of syncope in most cases, but not of the high mortality rate in these patients. The latter seems to be mainly related to underlying structural heart disease and ventricular tachyarrhythmias. Unfortunately, EPS does not seem to be able to correctly identify the high-risk patients and the finding of inducible ventricular arrhythmias should be interpreted with caution.

Suspected tachycardias

Supraventricular tachycardias

Paroxysmal supraventricular tachycardia (PSVT) should be suspected in patients with syncope and palpitations in the absence of structural heart disease. PSVT presenting as syncope without accompanying palpitations is relatively rare, but can occur at the onset of an attack or just after its termination when a pause may ensue before normal sinus function is restored. Transesophageal pacing, as well as invasive EPS with and without pharmacologic challenge (usually individually titrated doses of parenteral isoproterenol and/or atropine), may be used to both facilitate induction of PSVT and evaluate the hemodynamic effects of tachycardia. In either case, it is usually necessary to position the patient in an upright posture (e.g., using a tilt-table) in order to recognize the full hemodynamic impact of the arrhythmia.

Recognition of PSVT as a cause of syncope is important, as many cases are curable by radiofrequency ablation. The most frequent curable PSVTs are: (i) re-entry within the AV node (AV node re-entrant tachycardia) (Figs 10.3 & 10.4); (ii) re-entry using an overt or concealed accessory AV pathway (e.g., WPW syndrome, or other AV re-entrant tachycardia); and (iii) atrial flutter (a usually due to a large re-entry loop within the right atrium). Ectopic atrial tachycardias may also be subject to cure.

Atrial fibrillation can be associated with syncope due to inadequate reflex vascular compensation at the onset of an episode, or to delayed return of normal rhythm at the termination of an episode. In cetain cases, especially WPW syndrome, syncope may occur due to exceptionally rapid ventricular rates (Figs 10.5 & 10.6). EPS in such patients may be useful to determine whether atrial fibrillation is occurring as a consequence of another treatable rhythm (e.g., PSVT), or is the primary problem itself. Primary atrial fibrillation can be treated by ablation in some patients, while in others ablation of the His bundle and placement of a cardiac pacemaker can be very effective in preventing excessively rapid syncope-inducing heart rates during atrial fibrillation.

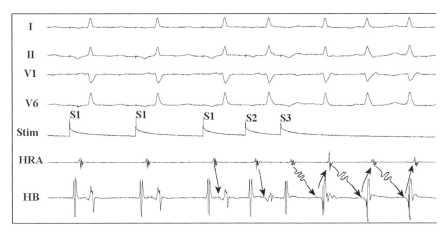

Fig. 10.3 ECG and intracardiac electrograms illustrating initiation of paroxysmal supraventricular tachycardias by placement of premature atrial beats (labelled S2 and S3) during EPS. From top to bottom the recordings are ECG leads I, II, VI and V6; intracardiac tracings are from the right atrium (labeled HRA) and the His bundle region (labeled HB). This tachycardia was determined to be due to AV node re-entry.

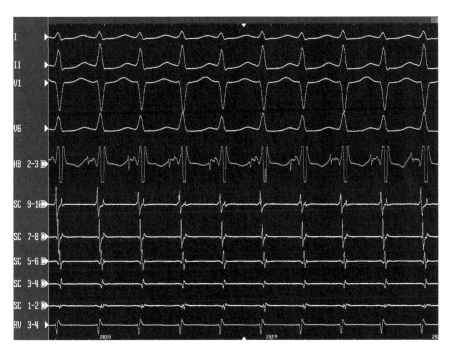

Fig. 10.4 Sustained paroxysmal supraventricular tachycardias. The ECGs and electrograms are as in Fig. 10.1. Note the His bundle potential in front of each ventricular electrogram on the HB channel. The atrial signals in all areas of the heart are almost simultaneous with the ventricular signals, strongly supporting a diagnosis of AV node re-entry.

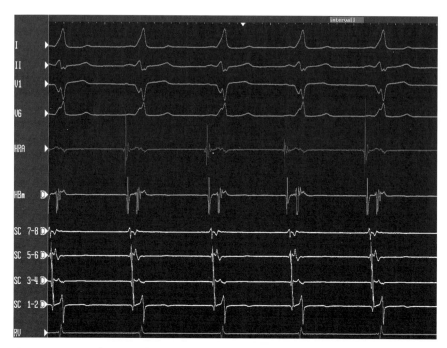

Fig. 10.5 ECG and intracardiac tracings in a patient with Wolff–Parkinson–White syndrome. Note the slurred upstroke of the QRS suggesting pre-excitation.

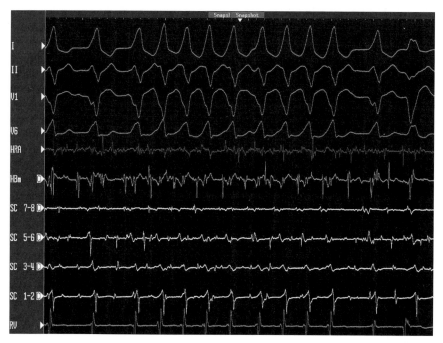

Fig. 10.6 Tracings during atrial fibrillation in the same patient as in Fig. 10.5. Note the very rapid and irregular ventricular response with QRSs of varying morphology depending on the degree to which AV conduction proceeded down the bypass connection versus the AV node. This rapid rate could cause hypotension with syncope, and in rare cases may degenerate into ventricular fibrillation.

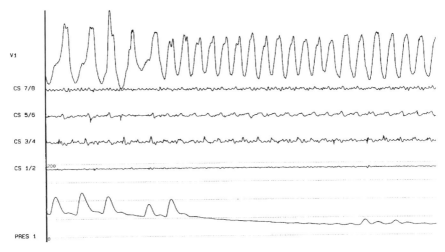

Fig. 10.7 Recordings illustrating onset of monomorphic ventricular tachycardia (VT) during EPS in a patient susceptible to recurrent hypotensive VT.

Finally, EPS may help to identify the infrequent patient in whom an atrial antitachycardia pacemaker or ICD can be helpful.

Ventricular tachycardias
Ventricular tachycardia may present as syncope with or without palpitations or other accompanying symptoms. With regard to syncope due to ventricular tachyarrhythmias, certain clinical features are useful to the clinician to suspect this possibility. The most important are:
- age;
- positive signal-averaged ECG;
- diminished left ventricular ejection fraction, and/or left ventricular aneurysm;
- history of myocardial infarction;
- coronary artery disease; and
- history of sustained monomorphic ventricular tachycardia on ambulatory ECG.

The major concern with programmed electrical stimulation as part of an EPS for inducing clinically significant ventricular arrhythmia is its varying sensitivity and specificity in different clinical settings and stimulating protocols. Generally speaking, programmed electrical stimulation is thought to be a sensitive tool (90–95%) in patients with chronic ischemic heart disease (previous myocardial infarction) and susceptibility for spontaneous monomorphic ventricular tachycardia (Fig. 10.7). Programmed electrical stimulation has a low predictive value in patients with non-ischemic dilated cardiomyopathy and most "primary" electrical disturbances in the setting of a relatively normal heart structure (e.g., long QT syndrome [Fig. 10.8]).

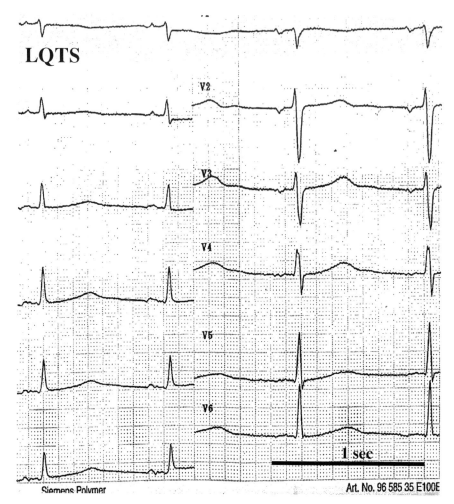

Fig. 10.8 12-lead ECG from patient with long QT syndrome. These patients are very prone to syncope due to susceptibility to torsades de pointes VT (see Chapter 14, Part 3).

In the ESVEM trial, a trial composed of ischemic heart disease patients, syncope associated with induced ventricular tachyarrhythmias during EPS indicated a high risk of death, similar to that in patients with documented spontaneous ventricular tachyarrhythmias. Polymorphic ventricular tachycardia and ventricular fibrillation, on the other hand, have previously been considered non-specific findings, a concept that probably needs modification depending on the clinical setting. One example is patients with Brugada syndrome in whom the induction of polymorphic ventricular arrhythmias seems to be the most consistent finding (Fig. 10.9).

The advent of ICDs with improved documentation of arrhythmic events offers a safe and sensitive tool for the follow-up (and thereby ultimately

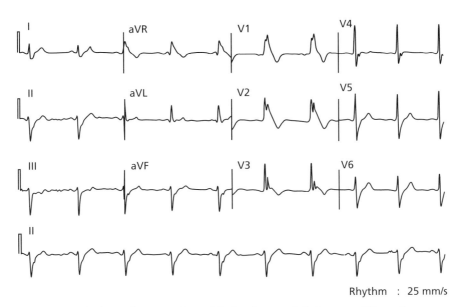

Fig. 10.9 12-lead ECG from a patient with the characteristic features of Brugada syndrome. Note the right bundle branch block appearance in V1, and the associated coved and elevated ST segment (see text for details).

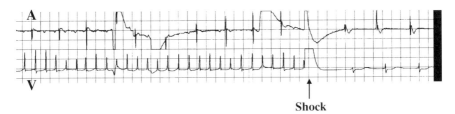

Fig. 10.10 Termination of an episode of VT by an ICD shock. The ICD terminates a life-threatening rhythm, but the patient may nonetheless experience syncope or near-syncope during the time it takes the device to detect the arrhythmia and charge the capacitors needed to deliver the shock.

better understanding) of potentially high-risk populations. The ESC syncope task force reviewed seven studies evaluating the utility of ICDs in a small number of highly selected patients with syncope (Fig. 10.10). In 67 patients with unexplained syncope and coronary artery disease (mostly with a prior myocardial infarction and ejection fraction of $37 \pm 13\%$), monomorphic ventricular tachycardia was induced in 43% of these patients. During > 1 year follow-up, 41% of the inducible patients received appropriate ICD therapy. ICD therapy was highly effective to prevent recurrence of syncope in these patients. However, the total mortality for patients with inducible monomorphic ventricular tachycardia was significantly higher than for non-inducible patients. The respective 1- and 2-year survival rates were 94% and 84% in non-inducible patients and 77% and 45% in inducible patients ($P = 0.02$), respectively.

It seems that patients with inducible ventricular tachycardia have similar incidence of ICD discharges (approximately 50%) compared with patients with previously documented spontaneous ventricular tachycardia at 1 year follow-up. A high correlation between recurrence of syncope and ventricular arrhythmias has been observed in patients with inducible ventricular arrhythmias (85%), similar to that in those with spontaneous ventricular arrhythmias (92%).

The predictive value of programmed electrical stimulation remains controversial in patients with unexplained syncope and non-ischemic dilated cardiomyopathy. In 14 patients with non-ischemic dilated cardiomyopathy, unexplained syncope and negative EPS, the incidence of appropriate ICD therapy is approximately 50% at 2 years follow-up, similar to that in patients with a documented cardiac arrest due to ventricular tachyarrhythmias (42%). The relapse of syncope or presyncope in these patients is primarily due to ventricular fibrillation. Finally, ICD therapy in these patients has been shown to be associated with improved survival.

Summary

EPS with programmed electrical stimulation is generally a helpful diagnostic test for patients with unexplained syncope but who have coronary artery disease and markedly decreased cardiac function. Its utility is more questionable for patients with non-ischemic dilated cardiomyopathy or valvular heart disease. EPS is of little diagnostic value in patients with normal hearts, in the absence of a documented (or at least strongly suspected) supraventricular or ventricular tachyarrhythmia.

In selected patients, EPS may be helpful in defining the nature and severity of an AV conduction disturbance, and the nature of an inducible tachycardia. In both settings such testing may help to define useful treatment strategies such as pacemakers, ICDs and ablation. With regard to ICD therapy, syncope patients with severe left ventricular dysfunction who undergo implantation of an ICD have a high incidence of appropriate spontaneous ventricular arrhythmia requiring antitachycardia pacing or shocks, suggesting that ICD therapy is effective for suppression of syncopal recurrences in this setting.

Further reading

Bigger JT Jr, Reiffel JA, Livelli FD, Wang PJ. Sensitivity, specificity, and reproducibility of programmed ventricular stimulation. *Circulation* 1986; 73 (Suppl II): 73–78.

Olshansky B, Hahn EA, Hartz VL, Prater SP, Mason JW. Clinical significance of syncope in the electrophysiologic study vs. electrocardiographic monitoring (ESVEM) trial. *Am Heart J* 1999; 137: 878–886.

Englund A, Bergfeldt L, Rehnqvist N, Åström H, Rosenqvist M. Diagnostic value of programmed ventricular stimulation in patients with bifascicular block: a prospective study of patients with and without syncope. *J Am Coll Cardiol* 1995; 26: 1508–1515.

Link M, Kim KM, Homoud M, Estes III M, Wang P. Long-term outcome of patients with syncope associated with coronary artery disease and a non-diagnostic electrophysiological evaluation. *Am J Cardiol* 1999; 83: 1334–1337.

Gaggioli G, Bottoni N, Brignole M *et al.* Progression to second or third-degree atrioventricular block in patients electrostimulated for bundle branch block: a long-term study. *G Ital Cardiol* 1994: 24: 409–416.

Fonarow GC, Feliciano Z, Boyle NG *et al.* Improved survival in patients with non-ischemic advanced heart failure and syncope with an implantable cardioverter-defibrillator. *Am J Cardiol* 2000; 85: 981–985.

Knight BP, Goyal R, Pelosi F *et al.* Outcome of patients with non-ischemic cardiomyopathy and unexplained syncope treated with an implantable defibrillator. *J Am Coll Cardiol* 1999; 33: 1964–1970.

Moya A, Brignole M, Menozzi C, Garcia-Civera R, Tognarini S, Mont L, Botto G, Giada F, Cornacchia D, and ISSUE Investigators. Mechanism of syncope in patients with isolated syncope and in patients with tilt-positive syncope. *Circulation* 2001; 104: 1261–1267.

Brignole M, Menozzi C, Moya A *et al.* The mechanism of syncope in patients with bundle branch block and negative electrophysiologic test. *Circulation* 2001, 104: 2045–2050.

Menozzi C, Brignole M, Garcia-Civera R *et al.* Mechanism of syncope in patients with heart disease and negative electrophysiologic test. *Circulation* 2002; 105: 2741–2745.

CHAPTER 11

Additional diagnostic testing for selected syncope patients

Lennart Bergfeldt, David G Benditt, Piotr Kulakowski, Michele Brignole

Introduction

In a patient with syncope the presence of structural heart disease and/or findings indicative of risk for life-threatening ventricular arrhythmias has important prognostic and therapeutic implications. It is against this background that this chapter reviews certain additional diagnostic tests that have potential value in selected patients. In this regard, echocardiography is relatively widely used to assess the nature and severity of suspected underlying structural heart disease. Other procedures such as exercise testing, coronary angiography and signal-averaged electrocardiography (ECG) have more limited applications.

Goals

The goals of this chapter are to review the indication for and utility of a number of diagnostic procedures designed to assess the nature and severity of underlying structural heart disease in the setting of the syncope evaluation. The following techniques are addressed:
- echocardiography;
- exercise testing;
- coronary angiography;
- heart rate variability;
- ATP (adenosine) test; and
- signal-averaged ECG.

Echocardiography

Echocardiography is frequently used as a screening test to detect and/or quantify the severity of cardiac disease in patients with syncope. Although numerous published case reports have suggested an important role of echocardiography in disclosing the cause and/or mechanism of syncope, larger studies have shown that the diagnostic yield from echocardiography is low in the absence of clinical, physical or ECG findings suggestive of a cardiac abnormality. However, even if echocardiography alone is only seldom diagnostic, this test may provide useful information regarding the type and severity of underlying heart disease; such findings may be helpful for risk stratification. If moderate to severe structural heart disease is found, evaluation is directed toward a cardiac cause of syncope. On the other hand, in the presence of minor structural abnormalities detected by echocardiography, the probability of a cardiac cause of syncope is less, and the evaluation may proceed as in patients without structural heart disease (see Chapter 4).

Echocardiography should be part of the initial evaluation when cardiac disease is suspected and/or when syncope is provoked by exercise, no matter the age of the patient. Identification of the presence and severity of structural heart disease is most effectively accomplished in this manner. In particular, estimation of left ventricular ejection fraction is essential in the presence of cardiac disease, particularly in those circumstances in which the therapeutic strategy may include a decision regarding use of antiarrhythmic agents or implantation of an ICD. In the former case, proarrhythmic and/or negative inotropic effects of certain drugs preclude their use in the setting of structural heart disease. In the case of ICD therapy, ejection fraction plays a major role in determining which patients are appropriate ICD candidates.

Apart from being of value in identifying patients with probable ischemic heart disease (i.e., regional wall motion disturbances) and significant valvular disease, echocardiography may suggest the presence of less common conditions which can be associated with syncope. Certain of these include hypertrophic cardiomyopathy with or without left ventricular outflow tract obstruction (HOCM, HCM), intracardiac tumors and pulmonary hypertension. In arrhythmogenic right ventricular dysplasia (ARVD), echocardiography may suggest the presence of the problem, but it is not nearly as sensitive as is magnetic resonance imaging (MRI) or preferably cine-MRI. With regard to ischemic heart disease, echocardiographic diagnostic sensitivity is enhanced by exercise or dobutamine stress.

Valvular heart disease not identified through the history or by the initial physical examination is probably rare. Nevertheless, certain conditions such as mitral stenosis and aortic stenosis may be unappreciated even by skilled examiners, and their relevance to patient symptoms only becomes evident after imaging assessment. In the case of aortic stenosis, syncope may occur for a variety of reasons including inadequate cardiac output during exertion, neurally mediated reflex events (similar to the vasovagal faint), and ventricular arrhythmias. Echocardiographic quantification of disease severity is far more precise than can be achieved by physical examination alone. Finally, intracardiac tumors (e.g., atrial myxoma) may only become evident by echocardiographic examination.

A normal echocardiogram is probably more helpful in the diagnostic evaluation of the middle-aged and older syncope patient, than in the young. In the latter group, neurally mediated reflex faints are the predominant cause of syncope, and these types of syncope are usually unassociated with structural heart disease. On the other hand, in rare cases echocardiographic examination may detect abnormalities of the origin of the coronary arteries (although the imaging procedure must be undertaken with that concern in mind), providing a potential explanation for exercise-induced symptoms.

Exercise testing

Exercise testing is not usually indicated in the evaluation of syncope, and is not particularly cost-effective when used in a general population with syncope. Its diagnostic yield was less than 1% in a population study. However, when its use is limited to selected patients with exertional syncope, it may represent an important diagnostic test. In such settings, the exercise test should always be symptom limited, and ECG and blood pressure recording should be extended throughout the recovery phase.

Exercise testing has a place in the evaluation of syncope that occurs during or in the immediate recovery phase after strenuous physical activity. Atrio-ventricular (AV) block may be provoked as the atrial rate exceeds the ability of the AV conduction system to sustain conduction—a rare finding, but with specific prognostic importance. When it occurs, it is usually in a patient with bundle branch block at rest, and is an ominous sign of transient or impending high-degree AV block. Progression to complete AV block is a concern in this setting. Resting ECGs in patients exhibiting exercise-induced AV block frequently show an intraventricular conduction abnormality, but not always. Coronary artery disease may be a contributory factor to exercise-induced AV block, and warrants further investigation.

Apart from identifying ST segment changes suggestive of ischemia or exercise-induced AV block, the heart rate response during exercise provides potentially useful additional information. Chronotropic incompetence observed during exercise may help to explain exertional lightheadedness or syncope. Chronotropic incompetence is part of the spectrum of sinus node disease. Various criteria for chronotropic incompetence have been suggested, but as a rough guideline a heart rate > 135 beats/min should be reached at maximum workload in the absence of treatment with negative chronotropic drugs. Further, its identification may signal the presence of other manifestations of sinus node dysfunction (e.g., sinus pauses), although sensitivity of such a test finding is probably low.

For patients treated with class IC antiarrhythmic drugs (flecainide, propafenone, etc.) widening of the QRS during exercise might signal a propensity for proarrhythmia. Occasionally exercise-induced repolarization abnormalities might disclose previously unrecognized long QT syndrome. Finally, in the presence of heart disease, and occasionally even in otherwise healthy persons, maximal or even supramaximal exercise testing might provoke ventricular arrhythmia, a potentially critical observation of a life-threatening nature.

Coronary angiography

Coronary angiography is seldom necessary in the syncope evaluation, and is rarely indicated to establish a diagnosis of coronary artery disease (since non-invasive methods are highly effective). Nonetheless, angiography has an obvious place when myocardial ischemia is believed to play a role in the syncopal attack, and in decisions related to the need for and feasibility of coronary revascularization.

Signal-averaged ECG, heart rate variability, QT dispersion and alternans

These tests have very limited utility in the syncope evaluation, and should only need to be ordered very infrequently. In general the use of these tests is intended to identify those patients with syncope in whom ventricular tachycardia may be the underlying mechanism and consequently are at high risk of sudden death. Nevertheless they are hampered by low positive predictive value. They are primarily reserved for the occasional syncope patient in whom other studies have identified the presence of ischemic heart disease, but additional risk stratification for sudden death risk is desired. In this regard, once it has been shown that a syncope patient has poor left ventricular function, it is not clear that these tests alter treatment decisions. For instance, it is unlikely that a negative signal-averaged ECG improves the prognosis in such a patient. Consequently, at least at the present time, most patients with this clinical profile will receive an ICD. Alternatively, where clinical history and examination and the resting ECG and echocardiogram are normal, it is unlikely that these tests are warranted as these patients have a good prognosis. However, if there is a family history of sudden cardiac death, despite an apparently normal echocardiographic assessment of left and right ventricular function, risk stratification tests may be useful in guiding a decision about treatment. An exception may be in patients with ventricular arrhythmias with left bundle branch block pattern. In such cases, the signal-averaged ECG might assist in the differentiation between ARVD and right ventricular outflow tract arrhythmia in the absence of structural heart disease, information that has prognostic implications and might affect the choice of therapy.

The ATP test

The value of bolus administration of ATP (or in some countries adenosine) remains a controversial topic. It has been suggested that the ATP test is a useful way of identifying a form of syncope associated with paroxysmal AV block in certain older individuals in whom other causes have been excluded. This suggests that ATP bolus administration might actually unmask occult AV nodal disease in susceptible individuals, and guide a decision to initiate permanent pacing.

The protocol proposed by Flammang *et al.* consists of the injection in a brachial vein of a bolus (< 2 sec) of 20 mg of ATP or adenosine (although ATP is by far preferred) followed by a 20-mL flush of dextrose solution or saline solution. During injection, patients remain supine with continuous ECG recordings just before and 2 min after drug administration. Blood pressure is monitored non-invasively. Due to possible bronchospastic reactions, ATP test is contraindicated in patients with known asthma. Interpretation of the result of the test is exclusively based on the duration of the cardiac pause; pauses > 10 sec, even if interrupted by some escape beats, are defined as abnormal (although some reports suggest that a pause > 6 sec is sufficient). In patients with abnormal responses, reproducibility was approximately 80% in both the short- and long-term period.

ATP testing produces an abnormal response in some patients with syncope of unknown origin, but not in controls. The diagnostic and predictive value of the test remains to be confirmed by prospective studies. In the absence of sufficient hard data, the test may be indicated at the end of the diagnostic work-up. The positive ATP test may prove to be an important marker for the need of a permanent pacemaker.

Summary

This chapter has examined certain ancillary diagnostic tests which may be useful in the evaluation of syncope patients. However, with the exception of the echocardiogram and possibly the ATP test, most of these studies have limited utility and poor diagnostic yield. They are only infrequently indicated, and their routine use is to be discouraged. The ATP test is currently undergoing further clinical evaluation in the US. Ultimately it may have a valuable role in selected older syncope patients.

Further reading

Kuchar DL, Thorburn CW, Sammel NL. Signal averaged electrocardiogram for evaluation of recurrent syncope. *Am J Cardiol* 1986; 58: 949–953.

Gang ES, Peter T, Rosenthal ME, Mandel WJ, Lass Z. Detection of late potentials on the surface electrocardiogram in unexplained syncope. *Am J Cardiol* 1986; 58: 1014–1020.

Steinberg JS, Prystowsky E, Freedman RA *et al.* Use of the signal-averaged electrocardiogram for predicting inducible ventricular tachycardia in patients with unexplained syncope: relation to clinical variables in a multivariate analysis. *J Am Coll Cardiol* 1994; 23: 99–106.

Sakaguchi S, Shultz JJ, Remole SC, Adler SW, Lurie KG, Benditt DG. Syncope associated with exercise, a manifestation of neurally mediated syncope. *Am J Cardiol* 1995; 75: 476–481.

Calkins H, Seifert M, Morady F. Clinical presentation and long-term follow-up of athletes with exercise-induced vasodepressor syncope. *Am Heart J* 1995; 129: 1159–1164.

Ascheim DD, Markowitz SM, Lai H, Engelstein ED, Stein KM, Lerman BB. Vaso-depressor syncope due to subclinical myocardial ischemia. *J Cardiovasc Electrophysio*l 1997; 8: 215–221.

Hattori R, Murohara Y, Yui Y, Takatsu Y, Kawai C. Diffuse triple-vessel coronary artery spasm complicated by idioventricular rhythm and syncope. *Chest* 1987; 92: 183–185.

Flammang D, Church T, Waynberger M, Chassing A, Antiel M. Can adenosine 5′ triphosphate be used to select treatment in severe vasovagal syndrome? *Circulation* 1997; 96: 1201–1208.

Brignole M, Gaggioli G, Menozzi C *et al*. Adenosine-induced atrioventricular block in patients with unexplained syncope. The diagnostic value of ATP test. *Circulation* 1997; 96: 3921–3927.

Flammang D, Erickson M, Mc Carville S, Church T, Hamani D, Donal E. Contribution of head-up tilt testing and ATP testing in assessing the mechanisms of vasovagal syndrome. Preliminary results and potential therapeutic implications. *Circulation* 1999; 99: 2427–2433.

CHAPTER 12

Neurologic diagnostic procedures in syncope

J Gert van Dijk

Introduction

In the context of transient loss of consciousness, neurologic diagnostic tests may be directed at four different fields—cortical function, structural integrity of the brain, the arteries supplying the brain, and the autonomic nervous system. Corresponding tests for the first three fields are the electroencephalogram (EEG), computed tomography (CT) and magnetic resonance imaging (MRI) scanning, and ultrasound investigation of the carotid and vertebral arteries. There is a wide range of tests to investigate the autonomic nervous system, of which the tilt-table test and tests of cardiovascular reflexes are most widely used.

The decision regarding which test to order and when, depends on the circumstances of specific attacks. For this reason, a careful history is without doubt the single most important procedure. The testing strategy should be based on the pattern of clinical presentation as discussed below.

Goals

The goals of this chapter are to:
- outline the role of neurologic studies in the diagnostic assessment of syncope; and
- examine appropriate evaluation steps in certain specific neurologic conditions that may cause syncope or syncope-like states.

Laboratory testing in the evaluation of syncope: an overview

In the evaluation of true syncope (defined as a transient, short-lived and self-limited loss of consciousness due to insufficient cerebral blood flow), there is no reason to order an EEG, CT, MRI or ultrasound investigation of the arteries supplying the brain. Unfortunately, numerous even very recent studies on syncope suffer from using a much less strict definition, in which no pathophysiologic mechanism is stated. The result is that entities such as concussion and seizures may end up in a "syncope" group. In such cases, the diagnostic strategy is then obviously different.

If one's intention is to encompass within the evaluation a broad array of conditions which may cause loss of consciousness, but are not just "syncope", then in order to prevent confusion it is best to use the phrase "transient loss of consciousness" (see also Chapter 17). This phrase incorporates a range of conditions and can be used until a likely cause has been established, such as syncope, epilepsy or concussion.

Readers may feel that they need a battery of tests precisely to make the distinction among various conditions which cause transient loss of consciousness, but this is rarely the case. The clinical presentation usually provides enough clues to choose among the main categories. Additional tests should be directed at disorders within the appropriate category. For example, in a patient with exercise-dependent attacks of unconsciousness and antecedent heart disease syncope is very likely, and the "a priori" chances of epilepsy are so low that an EEG is very unlikely to change this view.

Testing in specific conditions

Autonomic failure

Syncope in autonomic failure can benefit from ancillary neurologic testing. In such patients, the faint may occur through an orthostatic hypotension mechanism as well as through postexercise hypotension. In autonomic failure the neurologic dysfunction is often not restricted to blood pressure regulation, so history-taking should include sexual function (impotence), sweating (dry skin, sometimes with patches of compensatory hyperhidrosis), bladder function (both incontinence and retention), gastrointestinal function (delayed stomach emptying, constipation, diarrhea) and pupillary function (blurred vision).

History-taking is also important to distinguish between three groups of autonomic failure. Primary autonomic failure encompasses degenerative diseases such as multiple system atrophy, pure autonomic failure and autonomic failure in the context of Parkinson's disease. Secondary autonomic failure concerns damage to the autonomic nervous system in the context of other diseases, such as diabetes, kidney and liver failure, and alcoholism. In the third group, autonomic failure occurs as a side-effect of medication. Likely culprits are antidepressants, antihypertensives, vasodilators and beta-adrenergic receptor blocking drugs. In this drug-induced group, autonomic failure may be restricted to orthostatic hypotension.

The differential diagnosis of autonomic failure is complex, and requires considerable expertise. The same holds for the application of cardiovascular or other tests of autonomic function. When the more obvious causes, such as diabetes and drug effects have been excluded, an expert opinion should be sought.

Syncope mimics

As discussed elsewhere in this volume (Chapter 17), a large number of conditions are often diagnosed as "syncope", but in reality they do not cause true syncope. Thus we use the term "syncope mimics". In this group of conditions, investigations should be chosen based on the "a priori" chance of the disorder in question.

Epilepsy

The EEG has a twofold role in the diagnosis of epilepsy. Firstly, by showing "epileptiform abnormalities" it may considerably increase the likelihood of epilepsy being present and being the cause of loss of consciousness spells. The detected EEG abnormalities have different weights depending on their nature: some, like "spike–wave" complexes provide hard evidence, whereas sharp waves and a variety of other waveforms carry considerably less weight. Secondly, their nature and location help to identify the specific type of epilepsy. For instance, a typical 3 per second run of large spike–wave complexes all over the brain points to "absence" epilepsy, whereas isolated temporal spike–wave complexes are more often seen in partial complex epilepsy.

In the vast majority of cases the EEG is recorded interictally. The chance of detecting abnormalities decreases with each successive EEG. Thus, it rarely pays to order another EEG if two or three previous ones were normal for epilepsy. Photic stimulation (flashing light), hyperventilation and sleep de-privation are procedures that increase the chances of finding epileptiform abnormalities. These abnormalities are highly specific, in that they occur in only about 1% of people without overt epileptic attacks. In some cases it may be necessary to obtain an ictal recording to prove or disprove epilepsy as a cause for attacks. This may be done with ambulatory EEGs on an outpatient basis, or by video and EEG observation in a dedicated center.

Brain imaging by CT or MRI is indicated in epilepsy to search for the cause of epilepsy rather than to establish epilepsy itself. Thus, structural abnormalities such as brain tumors may be detected. However, such scans should only be ordered when concrete evidence points to a neurologic disorder, such as probable epilepsy. For probable syncope these scans should be avoided in view of their exceedingly low diagnostic yield. The only exception is syncope due to primary autonomic failure, but here too there should be clinical evidence suggestive of the underlying neurologic abnormality other than just the occurrence of syncope.

Subclavian steal syndrome

Syncope-like attacks provoked by physical exercise of the arms point to a steal phenomenon (often termed "subclavian steal syndrome"). Apart from measuring blood pressure in both arms, ultrasound studies are indicated to search for a steal syndrome. Note that not all steal phenomena result in clinical symptoms, so it is wise to think twice whether or not an observed steal phenomenon is to blame for a specific attack.

Strokes and transient ischemic attacks

Transient ischemic attacks (TIAs) obviously need accurate diagnosis and prompt medical attention, but in the context of syncope it should be understood that they do not really look like syncope. In carotid TIAs, neurologic deficits such as hemiparesis or aphasia predominate while consciousness is normal. Only TIAs involving a very large proportion of the cortex can impair consciousness. However, even these do not usually go as far as complete loss of consciousness. Further, they last too long to look like syncope, and the deficit will be impressive. Vertebrobasilar TIAs are theoretically more likely to mimic syncope, but again loss of consciousness is not very common, and there are a large number of additional signs, such as dysarthria, ataxia, vertigo and nystagmus to suggest the diagnosis.

There is no need to order a CT scan, MRI or ultrasound studies of the carotid or vertebral arteries for attacks looking like syncope but in which the history and physical findings clearly point away from a structural neurologic problem, i.e., loss of consciousness without neurologic deficit.

"Hyperventilation syndrome"

This name was (and sometimes still is) used for attacks of anxiety together with a variety of somatic complaints, such as shortness of breath, a tight sensation in the chest and tingling fingers. It was built on the theory that hyperventilation induced hypocapnia, which induced cerebral vasoconstriction, leading to cerebral hypoxia and the complaints. However, subsequent studies have showed that the attacks also occurred in the absence of hypocapnia. Thus, the presumed pathophysiologic theory has been proved to be incorrect. This also means that the hyperventilation provocation test aiming for complaint recognition is dubious, as it is not clear what is being tested. Attacks of a similar nature fall under the term "panic attacks" in the psychiatric nomenclature.

Summary

Neurologic disease is rarely the cause of true syncope, although it may cause periods of transient impairment of consciousness or seemingly transient impairment of consciousness which can be mistaken for syncope (e.g., epilepsy). Consequently neurologic testing is rarely indicated in the diagnostic evaluation of the cause of syncope. Such testing should not be part of the initial assessment of syncope patients. For those patients suspected of primary autonomic failure or epilepsy, referral to a neurologic specialist is warranted.

Further reading

Flink R, Pedersen B, Guekht AB *et al.* Guidelines for the use of EEG methodology in the diagnosis of epilepsy. International League Against Epilepsy: commission report. Commission on European Affairs: Subcommission on European Guidelines. *Acta Neurol Scand* 2002; 106: 1–7.

Hornsveld HK, Garssen B, Dop MJ, van Spiegel PI, de Haes JC. Double-blind placebo-controlled study of the hyperventilation provocation test and the validity of the hyperventilation syndrome. *Lancet* 1996; 348: 154–158.

CHAPTER 13

Contribution of psychiatric disorders to apparent syncope

George Theodorakis

Introduction

Psychiatric disorders are known to be associated with and possibly responsible for certain "apparent" loss of consciousness episodes. However, a causal relationship should not be accepted easily. In fact, although psychiatric disturbances may be an important source of syncope mimics (see Chapter 17), they do not for the most part cause true syncope.

Goals

The goals of this chapter are to:
- identify the possible roles psychiatric disease may play in patients with apparent syncope; and
- review psychiatric conditions which may result in behavior that mimics syncope (pseudo-syncope).

In terms of the relationship between potentially abnormal psychiatric states and apparent loss of consciousness, several clinical scenarios may be relevant. First, syncope of "unknown etiology" may occur in patients who happen to have a coexisting psychiatric disorder. Most of these cases are probably vasovagal faints. Nevertheless, careful evaluation is needed. Syncope of any etiology may occur in such a patient population. Second, syncope-like episodes or syncope mimics are particularly common in association with certain psychiatric conditions (see later). In these cases it is important to keep the definition of syncope in mind (see Chapter 1). In the absence of cerebral hypoperfusion true syncope is not present, and anything else suggesting transient reversible loss of consciousness is then a mimic (see Chapter 17). Recognition is based on documenting that blood pressure and heart rate remain stable during the attack. Syncope in association with hyperventilation is a special case in which anxiety disorders and other psychiatric states might possibly be responsible for true syncope. Finally, psychiatric disorders may develop as a consequence of recurrent syncope episodes. In these cases, the recurring medical problem may be considered to be the source. However, proof of this relationship is difficult, and may only be possible after successful control of recurrent syncope ultimately results in resolution of the abnormal psychiatric state.

Association of syncope and psychiatric illness

In attempting to assess reports of an association between syncope and psychiatric diagnoses it is important to bear in mind that most studies use the term "syncope" more loosely than is used in this volume or is advised by the ESC Syncope Task Force. Thus, most published reports are difficult to assess as they almost certainly include both true syncope and syncope mimics.

Given the important caveat noted above, it is possible to get only a relatively uncertain sense of the psychiatry–syncope relationship. In this regard, in a study of the association between apparent syncope and psychiatric illness by Kapoor *et al.*, 163 patients suffering from recurrent unexplained syncope episodes were subjected to a diagnostic interview schedule (DIS). The DIS suggested a psychiatric diagnosis in 24.5%, with major depression in 12.3% and somatization, panic or anxiety disorders in another 14.7%. Compared with syncope patients in whom the cause of the faints were of known etiology, patients with syncope of unknown origin had higher rates of psychiatric disorders. This was especially true of panic disorders. Furthermore, patients with any psychiatric disorder had a 35% 1-year recurrence rate for syncope compared to 15% in those without a psychiatric disorder.

Similar conclusions have been reported by Linzer *et al.*, who found psychiatric disorders, in particular panic disorders and major depression, to be a common cause of syncope in 24–31% patients with "unknown etiology" syncope. Most of those patients exhibited positive head-up tilt testing suggesting that vasovagal syncope may have been the predominant underlying mechanism. However, these findings are subject to the concern that the conditions may be coexisting morbidities (or even laboratory false positives) rather than a causal relationship. It will be necessary to revisit this presumptive diagnosis in the future with more definitive diagnostic tools.

In a study by Kouakam *et al.*, psychiatric disorders were more frequent in patients with syncope in a cohort of 40 patients. Twenty-six patients (65%) had at least one psychiatric disorder compared to 14 (35%) control subjects. In the same study the psychiatric illness did not differ between positive and negative tilt test patients. Tilt testing was positive for vasovagal syncope in 63%. It was interesting that the existence of psychiatric disorder was a stronger predictor of syncope recurrence than tilt test result.

A wide range of disorders from simple emotional stress to psychiatric illnesses can be associated with syncope. However, it is uncertain whether these findings indicate a causal relationship. Central serotoninergic systems have been evaluated with clomipramine and other challenge drugs in patients with psychiatric disorders like major depression or panic disorders. Most of them have shown a significant increase in prolactin and cortisol in patients with panic disorders compared to normal controls, as a response to drug challenge.

These findings imply that an increased response to serotoninergic stimulus exists in these situations.

Evaluation of syncope patients with potential psychiatric contribution to symptoms

Medical history

As has been emphasized throughout this volume, a detailed medical history and a complete physical examination are essential in order to evaluate the possible contribution of psychiatric conditions to the evaluation of patients with apparent syncope. The history many times leads to the suggestion that a psychiatric component is present. For example, patients with multiple syncopal episodes without injury, or those who describe non-specific symptoms referable to many organ systems, lead one to think of psychogenic pseudo-syncope. This latter situation is usually related to psychologic factors causing the patients to manifest unexplained somatic symptoms. Of course, it is essential to evaluate the possibility of a "true" syncope diagnosis before labeling the disorder as psychogenic. The appropriate evaluation steps are described in other chapters in this volume.

Evidence from patients' relatives is useful. A preceding episode of anxiety, fear or various other somatic, stressful or panic phenomena with apparent hyperventilation, suggests a psychogenic cause (i.e., pseudosyncope). In the case of hyperventilation, "true syncope" may theoretically occur; the basis for this has been thought to be hypocapnia causing constriction of cerebral vessels and thus reduced cerebral blood flow. However, this mechanism is now less certain. In any case, it has not yet been clarified whether hyperventilation is a separate clinical entity or should be incorporated within the group of psychogenic causes of syncope.

Physical examination

The physical examination may be helpful in making the distinction between true syncope and pseudo-syncope. First, clinical examination during the syncope attack offers information regarding heart rate or blood pressure fall. In psychogenic pseudo-syncope, for example, the heart rate and blood pressure remain relatively stable during the attack. Sinus tachycardia may be expected. Second, in cases of psychogenic pseudo-unconsciousness, patients have a tendency to close their eyes when those are opened passively. The muscle tone of patients' limbs is also different than in real syncope. This results in a non-flaccid posture of the limbs in pseudo-syncope patients which is easily recognized by an experienced examiner. Likewise, the patient's hand when it is raised above the face and then released, will not drop on the face. Other signs include the observation that the eyes may show stable movements upwards or downwards, or consistently away from the observer.

Certain patients with psychiatric disease may appear to be unconscious for extended periods of time, unlike true fainters in whom the event is usually brief. In patients with prolonged periods of apparent pseudo-unconsciousness on a psychogenic basis, the real diagnosis may be overlooked and confused with syncope by some practitioners. However, the differential diagnosis should more reasonably consider coma rather than syncope.

Additional clinical considerations

Patients with vasovagal syncope frequently have somatization, anxiety, panic disorders or major depressive disorder. Psychiatrists often rely on the *Diagnostic and Statistical Manual of Mental Disorders* (i.e., *DSM IV*) to evaluate these patients. There are specific criteria that characterize individual psychiatric disorders.

Apart from the psychiatric component contributing to syncope, many patients suffering from psychiatric problems use drugs which may influence vascular tone and blood pressure, or which are potentially proarrhythmic. These should be taken into account as possible triggers of true syncope. Such drugs include phenothiazines, tricyclic antidepressants and monoamine oxidase inhibitors. QT interval prolongation, with susceptibility to torsade de pointes ventricular tachycardia is a major concern with several of these agents. Overdose is of course another concerning issue in this population. Revision of the patient's medications and/or ease of access to medications may solve the syncope problem.

Tests for psychiatric syncope patients

A number of tests may be useful in an attempt to identify patients with "psychiatric syncope". These include: (i) hyperventilation test; (ii) head-up tilt testing; (iii) electroencephalogram (EEG) or Doppler cerebral blood flow; and (iv) psychiatric diagnostic testing alluded to earlier.
- Hyperventilation test is performed with 3-min open-mouthed forced hyperventilation, and is considered useful. It has an estimated, but not well established, positive predictive value of 59% for diagnosing "psychiatric syncope" in young adults. This test is in need of additional study and is not yet widely accepted. Furthermore, since hyperventilation can provoke angina or heart block, vital signs should be monitored with continuous ECG recording.
- Tilt-table testing is widely used for evaluation of these patients. Most reactions observed are vasovagal (see Chapters 9 & 14, Part 1). However, there is often an overlap between vasovagal syncope and psychiatric illness. The tilt test can be performed without drug challenge or after provocation with isoproterenol, nitroglycerin, adenosine or perhaps other agents such as clomipramine.

Patients with psychosomatic syncope during head-up tilt testing show an apparent unconsciousness response with intact blood pressure and heart rate. Patients with such a response may warrant a thorough neurologic evaluation to exclude other causes of true unconsciousness. In such cases, further investigation with an EEG or cerebral blood flow could be useful (although not likely), but psychiatric assessment is certainly crucial.

Summary

A relation between psychiatric illness and apparent syncope-like states, especially affecting patients mainly with panic attacks, anxiety or depression, is quite common. Some have suggested that there is a "vicious circle" where syncope can lead to psychologic distress and dysfunction. On the other hand, vasovagal syncope can apparently result from anxiety and depressive disorders. In either case, the practitioner must carefully exclude causes of "true syncope" before concluding that the patient has a psychogenic disorder.

Further reading

Kapoor W, Fortunato M, Hanusa B, Schulberg H. Psychiatric illness in patients with syncope. *Am J Med* 1995; 99: 505–512.

Linzer M, Felder A, Hackel A *et al*. Psychiatric syncope: a new look at an old disease. *Psychosomatics* 1990; 31: 181–188.

Theodorakis GN, Markianos M, Livanis EG, Zarvalis E, Flevari P, Kremastinos DT. Hormonal responses during head up tilt-table test in neurally mediated syncope. *Am J Cardiol* 1997; 79: 1692–1695.

Theodorakis GN, Markianos M, Livanis EG, Zarvalis E, Flevari P, Kemastinos DT. Provocation of neurocardiogenic syncope by clomipramine administration during head-up tilt test in vasovagal syndrome. *J Am Coll Cardiol* 2000; 36: 174–178.

Kouakam C, Lacroix D, Klug D, Baux P, Marquie C, Kacet S. Prevalence and prognostic significance of psychiatric disorders in patients evaluated for recurrent unexplained syncope. *Am J Cardiol* 2002; 89: 530–535.

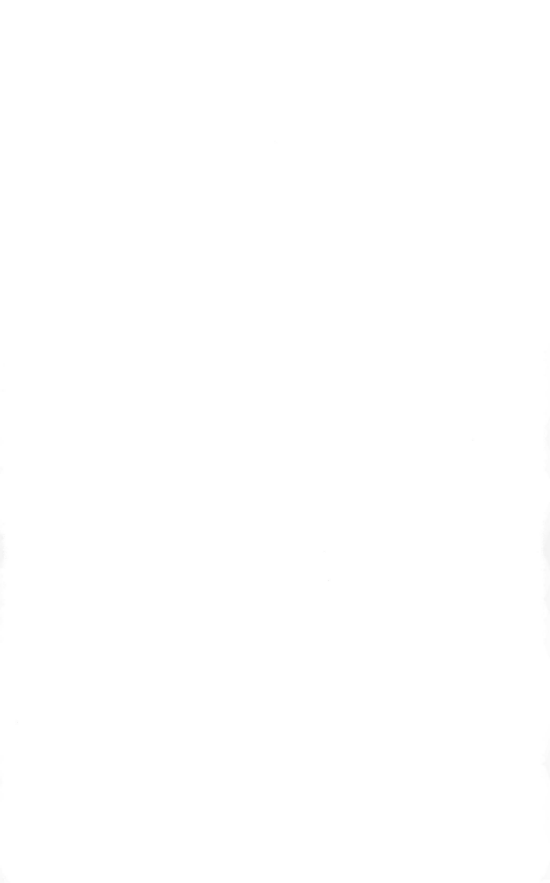

Section four:
Causes of syncope and syncope mimics, and treatment

Specific causes of syncope: their evaluation and treatment strategies

Part 1: Neurally mediated reflex syncope

David G Benditt, Jean-Jacques Blanc

Introduction

Neurally mediated reflex syncope (see also Chapter 1) encompasses a group of disorders, the best known forms of which are the vasovagal (or "common") faint and carotid sinus syndrome (Table 14.1). The former is generally believed to be the most frequent of all causes of syncope in humans. The latter (carotid sinus syndrome) has possibly been underappreciated as a cause of syncope and "falls". Postmicturition syncope, defecation syncope and cough syncope are probably the next most frequently occurring forms of neurally mediated faints. These latter conditions are often subclassified as so-called "situational" faints, since they are associated with specific scenarios (e.g., micturition, coughing, straining at stool).

Table 14.1 Neurally mediated reflex syncopal syndromes.

Common or "vasovagal" faint
Carotid sinus syncope
Situational faints
Postmicturition syncope
Cough, sneeze syncope
Defecation syncope
Postexercise variant
Swallow syncope
Glossopharyngeal neuralgia
Brass or wind instrument playing
Weightlifting

Goals

The goals of this part of the chapter are to:
- review the most common forms of neurally mediated reflex syncope and their diagnostic features;
- discuss the laboratory studies used to help establish the diagnosis; and
- provide a brief review of treatment options.

Evaluation

Medical history

The strategy for establishing a diagnosis of one of the neurally mediated reflex syncopes relies heavily on the obtaining of a detailed medical history. The reports of eye-witnesses are particularly important. The reader is referred to Chapter 5 for details regarding specific elements of the taking and interpreting of the medical history in these patients. Most important is the documentation of the details of patient activity, environment and symptoms immediately prior to the faint, and in the period following recovery. Witness observations of the event itself are also extremely valuable.

The vasovagal faint (also known as the "common faint") may be triggered by any of a variety of factors. In the case of the "classic" vasovagal faint these include unpleasant sights, pain, extreme emotion and prolonged standing. Consequently, circumstances surrounding a faint may lead to suspicion of vasovagal syncope as the cause. However, most informed practitioners have come to realize that the so-called "classic" features of vasovagal are more often than not either absent or not recollected. Therefore, even a detailed medical history undertaken by an experienced individual may not provide a definitive diagnosis. In such cases additional testing is prudent. Tilt-table testing is the most important readily available supportive test (see later).

Carotid sinus syndrome is the second most common form of neurally mediated syncope, but is often overlooked in clinical practice. "Spontaneous carotid sinus syndrome" may be defined as syncope which:
- by history, seems to occur in close relationship with accidental mechanical manipulation of the neck (and presumably the carotid sinuses); and
- can often be reproduced by carotid sinus massage (the role of neck muscle deafferentation as a contributing cause is also of importance, but that discussion lies beyond the scope of this chapter).

Spontaneous carotid sinus syndrome is rare and accounts for only about 1% of all causes of syncope. On the other hand, "induced carotid sinus syndrome", is more broadly defined, and may be accepted to be present even though a close relationship between manipulation of the carotid sinus and the occurrence of syncope is not demonstrated. Thus, induced carotid sinus syndrome is diagnosed when patients are found to have an abnormal response to carotid sinus massage and an otherwise negative work-up for syncope. Regarded in this way, carotid sinus syndrome is much more frequent, being found in 26–60% of patients affected by unexplained syncope. The occurrence of syncope or unexplained "falls", especially in older persons, should lead to consideration of carotid sinus syndrome.

Situational faints (e.g., postmicturition syncope, cough syncope, etc.) are diagnosed primarily by a careful history-taking. The "trigger" events surrounding the faints must be carefully searched for in the history-taking.

Laboratory studies

To date, the head-up tilt-table test is the only diagnostic tool to have been scrutinized to assess its effectiveness in the diagnosis of vasovagal syncope (see Chapter 9). Such testing, especially when undertaken in the absence of drugs, appears to discriminate well between symptomatic patients and asymptomatic control subjects. In fact, there is strong evidence to suggest that tilt-table testing at angles of 60–70 degrees, in the absence of pharmacologic provocation, exhibits a specificity of approximately 90%. In the presence of pharmacologic provocation, test specificity may be reduced, but nonetheless remains in a range that permits the test to be clinically useful.

Carotid sinus syndrome can also be assessed in the clinical laboratory, although the specificity and sensitivity of the carotid sinus massage procedure has not been rigorously studied. Nevertheless, based on consensus opinion, carotid sinus syndrome may be diagnosed when carotid sinus massage reproduces symptoms in conjunction with a period of asystole, paroxysmal atrioventricular (AV) block, and/or a marked drop (usually > 50 mmHg systolic) in systemic arterial pressure (see Chapter 9 for additional methodologic aspects). In many instances, the most convincing results from carotid sinus massage are obtained when massage is undertaken with the patient in the upright position (gently secured to a tilt-table for safety). Continuous arterial pressure and ECG recordings should be obtained throughout. The test is usually contraindicated if a carotid bruit is present or if the patient has symptoms suggestive of transient ischemic attacks. In the absence of symptom reproduction, a pause in the cardiac rhythm of 5 sec or longer is probably sufficient to support the diagnosis.

The situational faints are not readily assessed in the laboratory. Cough syncope may be an exception, but diagnostic criteria for hemodynamic response to induced cough have yet to be determined.

Treatment options

In general, initial "treatment" of all forms of neurally mediated reflex syncope comprises education regarding avoidance of triggering events (e.g., hot crowded environments, volume depletion, effects of cough, tight collars, etc.), recognition of warning symptoms, and maneuvers to abort the episode (e.g., supine posture, leg crossing). Additionally, if possible, strategies should address trigger factors directly (for example, suppressing the cause of cough in cough syncope). Specific thoughts regarding younger patients are found in Chapter 15.

Vasovagal syncope

In the vast majority of cases, patients who seek medical advice after having experienced a vasovagal faint require principally reassurance and education regarding the nature of the condition. Patients should be informed that vaso-vagal syncope is common in humans, and that in most people its occurrence is infrequent with only one or two events in a lifetime. However, certain indi-viduals have greater susceptibility, and multiple random recurrences are not uncommon in such cases. Initial advice should include review of the types of environments in which faints are more common (e.g., hot, crowded, emotion-ally upsetting, etc.), and provide insight into the typical warning symptoms (e.g., hot/cold feeling, sweaty, clammy, nauseated, etc.) which may permit many individuals to recognize an impending episode and thereby avert the faint. Thus, avoiding venipunture may be desirable when possible (e.g., not volunteering for blood donation), but psychologic deconditioning may be necessary. Additional common sense measures such as keeping well hydrated and avoiding prolonged exposure to upright posture and/or hot confining environments should also be discussed. With regard to these latter treatment concepts, formal randomized studies are not available.

When a more aggressive treatment strategy is needed, "volume expanders" (e.g., increased dietary salt and electrolyte intake with fluids such as "sport" drinks or salt tablets) or moderate exercise training appear to be among the safest initial approaches. Additionally, in highly motivated patients with recurrent vasovagal symptoms, the prescription of progressively prolonged periods of enforced upright posture (so-called "tilt training") may reduce syncope recurrence.

Many drugs have been used in the treatment of vasovagal syncope (beta-blockers, disopyramide, scopolamine, clonidine, theophilline, fludrocortisone, ephedrine, etilephrine, midodrine, clonidine, serotonin inhibitors, etc.). While the results have often been satisfactory in uncontrolled trials, placebo-controlled prospective trials have been unable to show a benefit of most of these drugs. The principal exception is midodrine, a vasoconstrictor agent.

Since failure of appropriate vasoconstriction of peripheral blood vessels is common to all of the neurally mediated reflex faints, vasoconstrictors may be employed. The new alpha-stimulating agents etilephrine and midodrine have both been studied in a placebo-controlled fashion. Etilephrine was studied as a segment of the randomized placebo-controlled VASIS trial, and proved to be ineffective. On the other hand, studies from Newcastle (UK) and Cleveland (USA) on short-term outcomes with midodrine in vasovagal syncope have shown a beneficial effect.

Head-up tilt laboratory findings have generally reported that pacing fails to prevent syncope, although it may prolong the premonitory warning phase. Nevertheless, unlike most other treatment avenues in this condition, pacing has been the subject of a number of both small single/multiple-center studies and major multicenter randomized controlled trials demonstrating effective-ness in select highly symptomatic patient populations. In this regard, the strongest supportive evidence comes from three randomized controlled trials: the North American vasovagal pacemaker study (VPS1), the European VASIS trial, and the SYDIT report. For example, in the case of the North American trial the actuarial 1 year rate of recurrent syncope was 18% for pacemaker patients and 60% for controls. The results of the pacing arm of the VASIS trial were similar; 5% of patients in the pacemaker arm experienced recurrence of syncope compared with 61% in the no-pacemaker arm during a mean follow-up of 3.7 years. However, these studies failed to account for the potential "placebo" effect of pacemaker implantation since unpaced patients did not have a device implanted. In this regard, the recently reported VPS2 trial suggests that when both groups (paced and not paced) undergo pacemaker implantation, the pacing benefit appears to be reduced in the first 6 months of follow-up. Whether the latter observation will change with longer follow-up remains to be seen. In the meanwhile, the SYNPACE study, in which all patients received pacemakers, may help to further clarify the value of pacemaker therapy, but has not been reported at this time.

Carotid sinus syndrome

Treatment of carotid sinus syndrome is in part guided by the results of the carotid sinus massage (i.e., relative importance of cardioinhibitory versus. vasodepressor responses; see also Chapter 9). Cardiac pacing appears to be beneficial in carotid sinus syndrome and is acknowledged to be the treatment of choice when bradycardia has been documented. For the most part, dual-chamber cardiac pacing is preferred. Medical therapy for carotid sinus syndrome has largely been abandoned.

The relationship between carotid sinus syndrome and spontaneous, otherwise unexplained, syncope has been demonstrated by pre/post comparative studies, two controlled trials, and a prospective observational study. Pre/post comparisons were done by analysing the recurrence rates of syncope in patients treated by pacing in several non-randomized studies. These studies show fewer recurrences at follow-up. Non-randomized comparative studies of patients receiving a pacemaker and untreated patients showed syncope recurrence rates to be lower in paced than non-paced patients. Brignole *et al.* undertook a randomized study in 60 patients; 32 patients were assigned to the pacemaker arm and 28 to the "no treatment" group. After a mean follow-up of 36 ± 10 months, syncope recurred in 9% of the pacemaker group versus 57% in the untreated patients ($p < 0.0002$). Finally, patients implanted with a pacemaker especially designed to monitor cardiac rhythm to detect asystolic episodes, showed long pauses (> 6 sec) in 53% after a 2-year follow-up, suggesting that a positive response to carotid massage predicts the occurrence of spontaneous asystolic episodes during follow-up.

As yet, there are no randomized studies examining treatment of carotid sinus syncope in which hypotension is predominantly of vasodepressor origin. Certain therapies used for vasovagal syncope may be expected to be of some benefit; vasoconstrictors and salt are the most likely in this regard, but the development of supine hypertension as a consequence of long-term treatment is a concern.

Situational faints

Treatment of most forms of neurally mediated situational syncope relies heavily on avoiding or ameliorating the trigger event. However, this may be difficult. For example, the "cough" trigger in cough syncope (for example, chronic obstructive pulmonary disease or asthma) is readily recognized, but suppressing it (the ideal treatment) is not easily accomplished. In other cases, avoidance of the "trigger" may have economic or avocation implications (e.g., syncope associated with blowing a wind instrument). In yet other cases, it is impossible to avoid exposure to the trigger situation (e.g., unpredictable emotional upset or painful stimuli, bowel movement in defecation syncope, bladder emptying in postmicturition syncope).

In conditions where trigger avoidance is not entirely feasible, certain general treatment strategies may be advocated. These include: maintenance of central volume; protected posture (e.g., sitting during micturition rather than standing); slower changes of posture (e.g., waiting after a bowel movement before arising); and recognition of increased risk when getting out of a warm bed. In specific conditions, certain additional advice may be helpful. Thus, use of stool softeners may help in patients with defecation syncope. Avoidance of excessive fluid intake (especially alcohol) just prior to bed-time may reduce risk in postmicturition syncope. Elimination of excessively cold drinks or large boluses of food may help in "swallow" syncope patients.

Guideline recommendations for treatment

Treatment is usually indicated when syncope or near-syncope:
- is accompanied by severe physical injury, or motor vehicle or other accident;
- occurs in a "high-risk" setting (e.g., commercial vehicle driver, machine operator, pilot, window washer, competitive athlete), or may result in substantial economic hardship, such as due to loss of employment or employment opportunity, or restricted lifestyle; or
- is sufficiently severe or frequent as to impair the patient's quality of life to a point which is unacceptable to the patient.

Treatment may sometimes be justified in patients with recurrent "falls", or "falls" associated with physical injury when clinical aspects suggest the possibility of a neurally mediated hypotension bradycardia (especially carotid sinus hypersensitivity) as a cause.

Treatment is not necessary in patients with single (or infrequent) syncopal episode(s), without injury and not in a high-risk setting and/or in which there are no over-riding economic or lifestyle concerns.

When a pharmacologic or pacemaker treatment is considered, a general prerequisite is to attempt to understand the relative importance of the cardioinhibitory and vasodepressor components of the reflex in causing syncope.

To do this the documentation of a spontaneous episode by means of ECG monitoring (including implantable loop recorder, ILR) or its provocation by means of carotid sinus massage or tilt testing is recommended.

Summary

Neurally mediated reflex syncope encompasses a wide variety of clinical scenarios. The vasovagal faint and carotid sinus syndrome are the most commonly encountered of these conditions but the various forms of situational faints are not rare. A detailed medical history is usually sufficient to obtain a diagnosis. Treatment may vary from education and reassurance, to physical maneuvers (e.g., leg crossing, tilt training) and finally drugs and pacemakers. The general physician, if confident of the diagnosis, should feel comfortable initiating the treatment program. Speciality referral is needed when the diagnosis is uncertain, or more aggressive therapy (e.g., drugs, devices) is thought to be necessary.

Further reading

Rushton JG, Stevens JC, Miller RH. Glossopharyngeal (vagoglossopharyngeal) neuralgia. A study of 217 cases. *Arch Neurol* 1981; 38: 21–205.

Kenny RA, Ingram A, Bayliss J, Sutton R Head-up tilt: a useful test for investigating unexplained syncope. *Lancet* 1986 June 14; 1: 1352–1355.

Almquist A, Goldenberg IF, Milstein S *et al*. Provocation of bradycardia and hypotension by isoproterenol and upright posture in patients with unexplained syncope *N Engl J Med* 1989 9; 320: 346–351.

Brignole M, Menozzi C, Gianfranchi L *et al*. A controlled trial of acute and long-term medical therapy in tilt-induced neurally mediated syncope. *Am J Cardiol* 1992; 70: 339–342.

Natale A, Akhtar M, Jazayeri M *et al*. Provocation of hypotension during head-up tilt testing in subjects with no history of syncope or presyncope. *Circulation* 1995; 92: 54–58.

Wieling W, Van Lieshout JJ, Van Leeuwen AM. Physical maneuvers that reduce postural hypotension in autonomic failure. *Clin Autonom Res* 1993; 3: 57–65.

Moya A, Permanyer-Miralda G, Sagrista-Sauleda J *et al*. Limitations of head-up tilt test for evaluating the efficacy of therapeutic interventions in patients with vasovagal syncope: Results of a controlled study of etilefrine versus. placebo. *J Am Coll Cardiol* 1995; 25: 65–69.

The Consensus Committee of the American Autonomic Society and the American Academy of Neurology. Consensus statement on the definition of orthostatic hypotension, pure autonomic failure, and multiple system atrophy. *Neurology* 1996; 46: 1470.

Ector H, Reybrouck T, Heidbuchel H, Gewillig M, Van de Werf F. Tilt training: a new treatment for recurrent neurocardiogenic syncope or severe orthostatic intolerance. *PACE* 1998; 21: 193–196.

Connolly SJ, Sheldon R, Roberts RS, Gent M, Vasovagal pacemaker study investigators. The North American vasovagal pacemaker study (VPS): A randomized trial of permanent cardiac pacing for the prevention of vasovagal syncope. *J Am Coll Cardiol* 1999; 33: 16–20.

Sutton R, Brignole M, Menozzi C *et al*. Dual-chamber pacing is efficacious in treatment of neurally mediated tilt-positive cardioinhibitory syncope. Pacemaker versus no therapy: a multicentre randomized study. *Circulation* 2000; 102: 294–299.

Kerdiet CTP, van Dijk N, Linzer M, van Lieshout JJ, Wieling W. Management of vasovagal syncope: controlling or aborting faints by leg crossing and muscle tensing. *Circulation* 2002; 106: 1684–1689.

Reybrouck T, Heidbuchel H, Van De Werf F, Ector H. Long-term follow-up results of tilt training therapy in patients with recurrent neurocardiogenic syncope. *PACE* 2002; 25: 1441–1446.

Specific causes of syncope: their evaluation and treatment strategies

Part 2: Orthostatic syncope

Angel Moya, Wouter Wieling

Introduction

Orthostatic faints are those associated with movement from a more gravitationally neutral position (e.g., supine position) to one in which gravitation tends to further diminish cerebral blood flow (e.g., upright posture). Thus, the orthostatic faint is most readily identified by a careful medical history in which the association with postural change is documented (i.e., syncope occurring shortly after moving from a lying or sitting to a standing position).

Although even healthy individuals may experience a tendency to orthostatic hypotensive symptoms when they stand up (e.g., transient "gray-out" or "black out"), the groups most susceptible to orthostatic syncope are:
- older frail individuals;
- patients with other underlying medical problems (e.g., diabetes, alcoholic neuropathy);
- persons who are dehydrated from hot environments, diuretics or inadequate fluid intake; and
- individuals taking certain commonly prescribed medications such as diuretics, antidepressants and antipsychotics, antihypertensives, beta-adrenergic blockers, and vasodilators like nitroglycerin and alpha-adrenergic blockers.

Goals

The goals of this part of the chapter are to review:
- pathophysiology and clinical features of orthostatic syncope;
- approach to diagnosis of orthostatic syncope; and
- treatment options for orthostatic hypotension and syncope.

Pathophysiology of orthostatic hypotension

Patients with orthostatic hypotension have an inability to maintain arterial blood pressure when standing up (Fig. 14.1). With a significant and persistent decrease in systemic pressure, characteristic features resulting from retinal and cerebral ischemia occur. These include visual disturbances ("gray-out" or "black-out"), lightheadedness, dizziness or even loss of consciousness (i.e., orthostatic syncope) (Fig. 14.1). Symptoms resulting from impaired perfusion of muscle tissue causing complaints such as pain in the neck region ("coat-hanger" distribution), lumbar pain and angina pectoris may also occur. Typically symptoms develop on standing and resolve on lying down.

A mismatch between intravascular volume and required cardiac output upon standing is a common cause of orthostatic hypotension (Table 14.2). In a minority of cases, however, orthostatic hypotension results not from volume depletion, but from impairment of autonomic reflexes required for maintaining blood pressure in the upright position. In these patients orthostatic hypotension is caused by impaired capacity of sympathetic nerves to increase vascular resistance. Increased downward pooling of venous blood and a

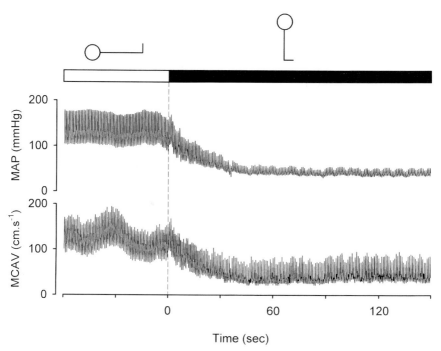

Fig. 14.1 Changes in blood pressure and cerebral blood flow in the middle cerebral artery in a 54-year-old patient with pure autonomic failure. Note marked drop of both pressure and flow with assumption of upright posture. (Reproduced after Harms *et al.* *Stroke* 2000; 31: 1608–1614 with permission of the editor.)

Table 14.2 Classification of orthostatic hypotension.

Volume depletion
Hemorrhage
Diarrhea
Salt-losing nephropathy
Addison's disease
Medications (diuretics)

Autonomic failure
Primary autonomic failure syndromes (e.g., pure autonomic failure, multiple system atrophy,
    Parkinson's disease with autonomic failure, acute pandysautonomia)
Secondary autonomic failure syndromes (diabetic neuropathy, amyloid neuropathy, chronic
    renal failure, alcohol, spinal cord transection, brain tumors)

Drugs
Sympatholytic medications (alpha-blockers, antidepressants)
Beta-adrenergic blockers

---

consequent reduction in stroke volume and cardiac output exaggerates the orthostatic fall in arterial pressure in these patients (Fig. 14.1). Autonomic failure can be due to a primary disease, secondary to other diseases that can affect the autonomic nervous system, or due to some drugs (Table 14.2).

Recent studies have reported that an abnormally large initial fall in blood pressure occurs in a variety of conditions that affect arterial baroreflex control of sympathetic activation of resistance vessels; for example, in patients with deafferented carotid sinus baroreceptors after neck surgery (impairment of afferent pathways), and in subjects receiving clonidine (blockade of central pathways). Symptomatic initial orthostatic hypotension is also reported to occur frequently in young subjects with a tendency to faint (see Chapter 15, Fig. 15.1), but the site of the lesion in the baroreflex arc in these subjects remains to be determined. The prevalence of inital orthostatic hypotension in elderly patients taking medications that are known to interfere with sympathetic function such as antidepressant and alpha-adrenergic blockers (Fig. 14.2) is unknown, but likely to be common.

Many elderly subjects are at risk of orthostatic hypotension because of age-related impairments in baroreflex-mediated vasoconstriction and cardioacceleration, as well as impaired diastolic filling of the heart. As a result of impaired diastolic relaxation, the aged heart often fails to generate an adequate stroke volume when preload is reduced as during upright posture.

Diagnosis

In elderly non-volume-depleted patients, in whom central or peripheral autonomic nervous system diseases have been excluded, orthostatic hypotension

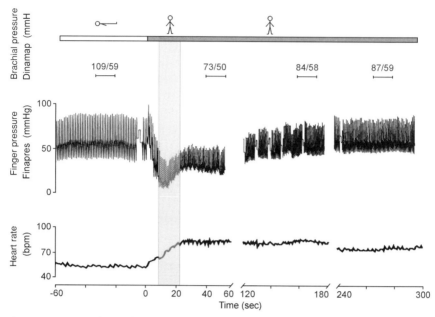

Fig. 14.2 Tracing obtained in a patient with recurrent unexplained syncope upon standing. Continuous monitoring of finger blood pressure documented an abnormally large transient initial fall in pressure accompanied by an appropriate compensatory increase in heart rate. The increased heart rate was unable to prevent substantial hypotension. A combination of medications known to impair orthostatic blood pressure control was responsible for the abnormality. (Revised after Wieling *et al. Clin Autonom Res* 2001; 11: 269–270 with permission of the editor.)

is prevalent in about 9% over the age of 80 and about 12% over the age of 85. It is a significant independent predictor of all-cause mortality.

Orthostatic syncope can be diagnosed when there is documentation of orthostatic hypotension associated with syncope or presyncope. Carefully measuring blood pressure with a sphygmomanometer supine and after standing suffices for the routine assessment of orthostatic blood pressure control in the office or at the bedside. For the diagnosis of orthostatic hypotension, arterial blood pressure must be measured when patient adopts the standing position after 5 min of lying supine. Orthostatic hypotension is defined as a decline in blood pressure of at least 20 mmHg systolic and/or 10 mmHg diastolic within 3 min of standing, regardless of whether or not symptoms occur. If the patient does not tolerate standing for this period, the lowest systolic blood pressure during the upright position should be recorded. Measurements should be continued after 3 min of standing if blood pressure is still falling at 3 min.

Initial orthostatic hypotension is difficult to assess with conventional measurement of blood pressure with cuff and stethoscope, as the blood pressure changes occur very rapidly (Fig. 14.2). Continuous non-invasive blood pressure measurement upon standing is needed to document this abnormality. However, in most cases the history will reveal that this condition is likely to be present.

There are some patients with syncope in whom there is a history suggestive of impaired orthostatic blood pressure control but in whom measurements in the upright position may be normal. In these patients additional tests after major provocative stimuli such as food ingestion and exercise may be needed to unmask orthostatic hypotension. A useful alternative is a 24-h or longer ambulatory blood pressure recording under daily living circumstances similar to those that are associated with symptoms in the individual patient.

The underlying diagnosis is of particular importance for patients with orthostatic hypotension. At the onset, it is important to identify non-neurogenic reversible causes of orthostatic hypotension like volume depletion, adrenal insufficiency (not common) and the effect of medications. The most frequent drugs associated with orthostatic syncope are vasodilators and diuretics. Alcohol can also be associated with orthostatic syncope, not only as a cause of orthostatic intolerance but also because it can induce autonomic and somatic neuropathy. Elimination of the responsible drug or offending agent is usually enough to improve symptoms. Reversible causes often coexist with neurogenic mechanisms and must be appreciated for optimal treatment, since they may substantially worsen orthostatic hypotension. Details of the diagnosis of primary and secondary autonomic disorders will not be discussed further here.

Treatment

Most experience of treatment of orthostatic hypotension failure has been obtained in patients with chronic primary autonomic failure, who have structural disorders with consistent failure of circulatory control and severe symptomatic orthostatic hypotension. By careful observation in these patients, valuable information has been obtained about the pathophysiology of abnormalities of orthostatic blood pressure regulation and its treatment (Table 14.3). Treatment strategies developed for patients with autonomic failure have been important for other patients with impairment of orthostatic blood pressure control.

General measures

The initial treatment in patients with orthostatic syncope includes advice and education about factors that can aggravate or provoke hypotension upon assuming the upright posture. These factors include avoiding sudden head-up postural change, especially on waking in the morning, standing still for a prolonged period of time, and straining during micturition and defecation. Other less common yet important considerations are hyperventilation, high environmental temperature (including hot baths, showers and saunas leading to dehydration with vasodilatation), large meals (especially with refined carbohydrates) and severe exertion. In addition, male patients with symptomatic

Table 14.3 General treatment principles and recommendations.

To be avoided
Sudden head-up postural change (especially on waking)
Standing still
Prolonged recumbence during daytime
Straining during micturition and defecation, hyperventilation
High environmental temperature (including hot baths and showers)
Severe exertion
Large meals (especially with refined carbohydrate)
Alcohol
Drugs with vasodepressor properties
Diet and cold preparations containing sympathomimetic amines

To be introduced
Salt intake of at least 8 g (150 mmol)/day
2–2.5 L fluid/day
Small frequent meals with a reduced carbohydrate content
Head-up sleeping
Judicious exercise (including swimming)
Physical counter maneuvers
Air-conditioning or fan in summer

To be considered
Abdominal binders
Elastic stockings
Support garment
Portable chairs

Pharmacologic treatment
Starting drug: fludrocortisone
Sympathomimetics: ephedrine or midrodrine
Specific targeting: desmopressin, erythropoietin, octreotide

orthostatic hypotension should also be advised to empty their bladders in a sitting position.

Iatrogenic factors are critically important in many orthostatic syncope patients. These are often older individuals who are being treated for a number of commonly occurring comorbidities such as hypertension, coronary artery disease and benign prostatic hyperplasia. As a result many such patients are prescribed drugs such as diuretics, vasodilators and beta-adrenergic and alpha-adrenergic blockers. Each of these can aggravate any predisposition to hypotension upon standing, and in some instances (e.g., excessive diuresis) may induce orthostatic symptoms.

Some patients with autonomic failure exhibit postprandial hypotension. In these patients, symptoms typically begin about 30 min after food ingestion and can last, even while supine, for up to 3 h. Carbohydrates appear to play a major role in causing hypotension. Alcohol can exert an additional effect by causing splanchnic vasodilatation. Consequently, these patients may improve by eating frequent smaller meals with reduced carbohydrate content and avoiding alcohol.

Patients with orthostatic hypotension should be encouraged to have a high dietary salt intake if there are no contraindications (e.g., concomitant hypertension or heart failure). At least 8 g of salt a day is advised by a liberal use of salt at mealtimes, by eating foods with a high salt content, or even with the use of salt tablets. Patients are advised to drink 2–2.5 L of fluids every day as well. Elderly patients may have a decreased sense of thirst and should in particular be encouraged to increase fluid intake. However, many tend to avoid fluids to prevent urinary frequency or incontinence.

Volume expansion can improve orthostatic tolerance markedly, with relatively small increases in arterial pressure (Fig. 14.3). This discrepancy between symptoms and the level of blood pressure can be explained by the fact that treatment shifts mean arterial pressure from just below to just above the critical level of perfusion of the brain. In patients with orthostatic hypotension in whom in spite of these general measures symptoms persist, several non-pharmacologic treatments can be applied.

Head-up sleeping at night

There is clear evidence that in patients with autonomic failure head-up sleeping increases the extracellular fluid volume and improves orthostatic tolerance, with improvement of symptoms. Two possible mechanisms that explain the effectiveness of this intervention have been suggested. Some authors have suggested that head-up tilt reduces renal arterial pressures and promotes renin release with consequent angiotensin II formation and aldosterone release that increases extracellular fluid and circulating blood. Other authors have suggested that with sleeping with the upper part of the body and head tilted upward ("head-up sleeping") there is an increase of the content of extracellular fluid volume in the lower extremities that leads to an increase in tissue pressure that prevents venous pooling. The fact that head-up sleeping became effective coincidentally with the appearance of slight edema in lower limbs supports this hypothesis. Effective head-up tilt sleeping can be achieved by elevating the head of the bed by 20–25 cm. To avoid sliding down while sleeping, a hard pillow under the mattress at the level of the buttocks can be used.

Physical countermaneuvers

In most patients with orthostatic intolerance, immobility can worsen symptoms, whereas bending forward, sitting or moving around can improve them. Based on these observations, several physical maneuvers that reduce venous pooling have been described (Fig. 14.4). The changes in blood pressure induced by these maneuvers can immediately be demonstrated to a patient by showing the finger blood pressure tracing on a video screen. Patients can

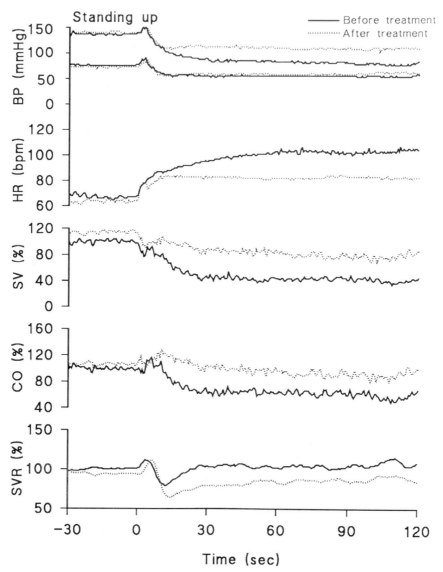

Fig. 14.3 Average heart rate, systolic and diastolic pressure, stroke volume, cardiac output and systemic vascular resistance responses to standing in six patients with autonomic failure before (continuous line) and after (dotted line) treatment with head-up sleeping, high salt diet and fludrocortisone medication. Blood pressure was measured with a Finapres device. Relative changes in stroke volume were computed by arterial pulse wave analysis. (From Ten Harkel *et al. J Int Med* 1992; 232: 139–145.)

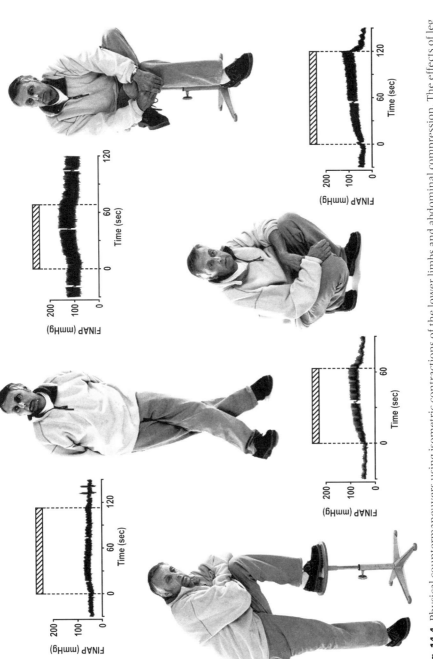

Fig. 14.4 Physical countermaneuvers using isometric contractions of the lower limbs and abdominal compression. The effects of leg crossing in standing and sitting position, placing a foot on a chair and squatting on finger arterial blood pressure (FINAP) in a 54-year-old male patient with pure autonomic failure and disabling orthostatic hypotension (same patient as Fig. 14.1). The patient was standing (sitting) quietly prior to the maneuvers. Bars indicate the duration of the maneuvers. Note the increase in blood pressure and pulse pressure during the maneuvers. (From Harms & Wieling, unpublished, with permission of the patient.)

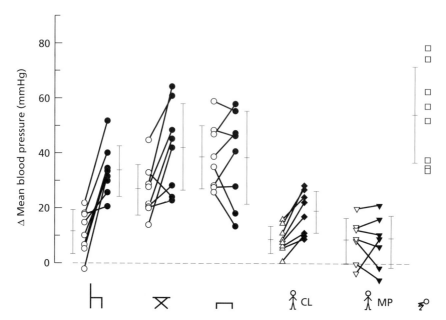

Fig. 14.5 The efficacy of sitting, crossing legs, muscle pumping and squatting to improve orthostatic hypotension in patients with autonomic failure. Mean finger arterial blood pressures are expressed as the blood pressure change during the intervention from the premaneuver standing blood pressure.

From left to right: sitting on a derby chair (height 48 cm), a fishing stool (height 38 cm) and a foot stool (height 20 cm), without (○) and with crossed legs (●); standing in crossed legs position (CL) without (△) and with (◆) contraction of lower extremity musculature; standing while muscle pumping (MP), marching on the spot (▽) and toe-raising (▼); and squatting (□). The vertical line represents mean and s.d. (Revised after Smit *et al. J Physiol* 1999; 519: 1–10 with permission of the editor.)

thereby be trained in applying the maneuvers effectively. Patients are advised to apply these maneuvers as soon as symptoms begin. However, for patients with motor disabilities or balance problems, these maneuvers can be difficult to apply.

Leg crossing

Crossing one leg over the other at thigh level while standing or sitting is an effective and easy maneuver that increases blood pressure. The beneficial effects of leg crossing have been attributed to mechanical compression of the venous vascular beds in the legs, buttocks and abdomen. Leg crossing has the advantage that it can be performed casually without much effort and without drawing attention to the patient's problem. Muscle tensing during leg crossing increases the beneficial effect of this countermaneuver on blood pressure considerably (Fig. 14.5).

Squatting

This is a highly effective maneuver that increases venous return rapidly and produces an important increase in systolic and diastolic arterial blood pressure (Fig. 14.5). It can be used as an emergency maneuver to prevent loss of consciousness when presyncopal symptoms develop rapidly. Bending over as to tie one's shoes has similar effects and is simpler to perform by elderly patients. In addition, sitting in the knee–chest position and placing one foot on a chair while standing, are comparable to squatting. When arising from the squatting position muscle tensing should be advised in order to prevent hypotension from recurring.

Bending forward

Lowering the head between the knees is a useful maneuver in fainting patients with autonomic failure. Lowering the head to the heart level is also a rapid way to enhance cerebral perfusion by decreasing the hydrostatic column between the heart and brain.

Skeletal muscle pumping

Maneuvers that use skeletal muscle pumping such as toe raising or repeated knee flexion have less reproducible effects in patients with autonomic failure, and as a consequence are clinically less effective (Fig. 14.5).

Additional measures

Other measures that decrease dependent pooling that can be used in patients with orthostatic hypotension include the use of portable folding chairs (Figs 14.4 and 14.5) and different types of pressure garments.

Pressor response to water drinking

Ingestion of a substantial amount of water is an intervention that is reported to be effective in combating orthostatic intolerance in patients with autonomic failure. After rapid drinking of about 0.5 L of water an increase in blood pressure is apparent within several minutes. The maximum effect (an increase of 20–30 mmHg on seated and standing systolic blood pressure) is reached after approximately 30 min and the effects are sustained for about 1 h (Fig. 14.6). For patients with autonomic failure the intervention is also effective to combat postprandial hypotension. Drinking of water also increases blood pressure substantially in healthy elderly, but not in healthy young subjects or patients with Parkinson's disease. The mechanisms underlying the rapid pressor response elicited by water drinking is debated. Sympathetic activation resulting in increased vasoconstrictor tone has been reported. Others have emphasized that the time course of the blood pressure response is unusually slow for sympathetic activation. These authors have suggested that minor elevations of intra- and extravascular fluid volume might be involved in patients with autonomic failure, who are extremely sensitive to changes in fluid balance. The

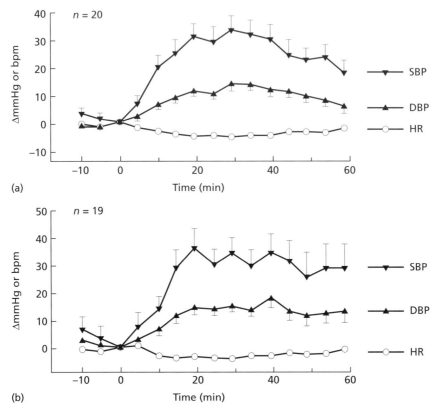

Fig. 14.6 Changes in systolic blood pressure (SBP), diastolic blood pressure (DBP) and heart rate (HR) induced by drinking of 480 mL of tap water in patients with multiple system atrophy (a) and pure autonomic failure (b). Patients started drinking at 0 min The blood pressure increase was evident within 5 min of drinking water, reached a maximum after approximately 20–30 min, and was sustained for more than 60 min. (From Jordan *et al. Circulation* 2000; 101: 504–509.)

afferent signal that activates the sympathetic system through water drinking remains to be fully elucidated.

Pharmacologic treatment
When non-pharmacologic treatments are not effective and symptoms persist, drugs are indicated. The most important of these drugs are described below.

Fludrocortisone
Fludrocortisone is the first drug of choice in the treatment of patients with autonomic failure. It is a potent synthetic mineralocorticoid with minimal glucocorticoid effect. It has several pharmacologic effects that can act in improving orthostatic blood pressure control in patients with autonomic failure. The

most important effect is an expansion of intravascular and extravascular body fluid. Other possible effects are a sensitization of vascular receptors to pressor amines and an increase in fluid content of vessel walls that increases their resistance to stretching. It is recommended to begin with a dose of 0.1 mg once a day, and it can be increased by 0.1 mg at 1–2-week intervals up to 0.3 mg daily, if needed. The pressor action is not immediate and takes some days to be manifest. The full benefit requires a high dietary salt intake. A weight gain of 2–3 kg is a reasonably good clue to adequate volume expansion. Mild dependent edema can be expected. Patients on fludrocortisone may develop hypokalemia within 2 weeks, and foods high in potassium such as fruits, vegetables, poultry, fish and meat should be advised. Occasionally potassium supplements may be needed. Headaches are another possible side-effect of fludrocortisone.

Midrodine

Midodrine is a prodrug that is converted to its active metabolite desglymidrodine after absorption. It acts on alpha-adrenoreceptors to cause constriction of both arterial resistance and venous capacitance vessels. It does not cross the blood–brain barrier and consequently does not have the undesirable central stimulant effects. Midrodine is administered in doses of 2.5–10 mg 3 times daily. Supine hypertension is a common side-effect. Midrodine may be of particular value in patients with severe postural hypotension and in those with peripheral lesions, as in pure autonomic failure. For unclear reasons, some patients on midrodine get worse. In such patients, there may be a reduction in intra- and extravascular fluid volume as manifested by weight loss.

Others

If the combination of fludrocortisone and sympathetic vasoconstrictor drugs does not produce the desired effect, selective targeting is then needed depending on the specific abnormality. Thus, desmopressin may be of value for patients with nocturnal polyuria, octeoride in those with postprandial hypotension, and erythropoietin in those with anemia. Such patients need to be referred to a specialized unit experienced in the use of these interventions.

Summary

Orthostatic hypotension is a common phenomenon as individuals move from a gravitationally neutral position to one in which they become more dependent upon vascular compensatory mechanisms to prevent hypotension and cerebral hypoperfusion. If a significant fall of systemic blood pressure occurs, orthostatic hypotension can lead to orthostatic syncope. The key factors affecting susceptibility to these types of faint include prescribed drugs, older age, dehydration and inadequate nervous system responsiveness (e.g., peripheral neuropathy). Treatment may be difficult, and relies on education, salt/volume replacement, physical maneuvers and drugs.

Further reading

Wieling W, van Lieshout JJ, van Leeuwen AM. Physical manoeuvers that reduce postural hypotension in autonomic failure. *Clin Autonom Res* 1993; 3: 57–65.

Smit AAJ, Halliwill JR, Low PA, Wieling W. Topical Review. Pathophysiological basis of orthostatic hypotension in autonomic failure. *J Physiol* 1999; 519: 1–10.

Omboni S, Smit AA, van Lieshout JJ, Settels JJ, Langewouters GJ, Wieling W. Mechanisms underlying the impairment in orthostatic intolerance after nocturnal recumbency in patients with autonomic failure. *Clin Sci* 2001; 101: 609–618.

Wieling W, Harms MPM, Kortz RAM, Linzer M. Initial orthostatic hypotension as a cause of recurrent syncope: a case report. *Clin Autonom Res* 2001; 11: 269–270.

Wieling W, van Lieshout JJ, Hainsworth R. Extracellular fluid volume expansion in patients with posturally related syncope. *Clin Autonom Res* 2002; 12: 243–249.

Jordan J. Acute effects of water on blood pressure—what do we know. *Clin Autonom Res* 2002; 12: 250–255.

Mukai S, Lipsitz LA. Orthostatic hypotension. *Clin Geriatr Med* 2002; 18: 253–268.

Schatz IJ. Orthostatic hypotension predicts mortality. Lessons from the Honolulu heart program. *Clin Autonom Res* 2002; 12; 223–224.

Goldstein DS, Robertson D, Esler M, Straus SE, Eisenhofer G. Dysautonomias: clinical disorders of the autonomic nervous system. *Ann Intern Med* 2002; 137: 753–763.

CHAPTER 14

Specific causes of syncope: their evaluation and treatment strategies

Part 3: Cardiac arrhythmias as a primary cause of syncope

Angel Moya

Introduction

Cardiac arrhythmias are an important cause of syncope. In some cases the arrhythmia may be secondary to other conditions, such as in the case of brady-arrhythmias associated with the various forms of neurally mediated reflex syncope (e.g., vasovagal syncope). These secondary circumstances are dealt with elsewhere in this volume. This section is devoted to those circumstances in which cardiac arrhythmias are thought to be the primary cause of symptoms. It details the most common arrhythmias to keep in mind when considering arrhythmia as the potential cause of syncope in an individual patient. The role of electrophysiologic study (EPS) is alluded to as part of this discussion (Table 14.4), but the reader is referred to Chapter 10 for a more a detailed analysis of the value and limitations of EPS in the syncope evaluation.

Goals

The goals of this part of the chapter are to:
- review the most common forms of syncope in which cardiac arrhythmias are the primary cause;
- provide an approach to establishing the specific diagnosis; and
- summarize clinical features of certain important but less frequent "arrhythmogenic" syndromes which are known to be associated with syncope.

Table 14.4 Minimal recommended electrophysiologic study protocol for assessment of syncope.

Measurement of sinus node recovery time (SNRT) and calculation of corrected SNRT by repeated sequences of atrial pacing for 30–60 sec each.

Assessment of AV node and His–Purkinje conduction (including HV interval measurement) at baseline sinus cycle length, and during atrial pacing at progressively faster rates until AV Wenkebach conduction is achieved. If these studies are inconclusive, and AV conduction disease remains suspected, the study should be repeated after infusion of antiarrhythmic drug unless contraindicated (ajmaline 1 mg/kg i.v. or procainamide 10 mg/kg i.v.).

Assessment of susceptibility to inducible supraventricular tachycardias by atrial extrastimulus testing (adding atropine and/or isoproterenol if necessary).

Assessment of susceptibility to ventricular tachyarrhythmias by ventricular extrastimulus testing at two RV sites, with two basic pacing frequencies, and employing up to two extrastimuli with progressively decreasing coupling intervals until ventricular refractoriness is achieved or the shortest coupling interval is 200 ms.*

---

*A third extrastimulus may be added to increase sensitivity, and occasionally infusion of isoproterenol is warranted. The latter are particularly warranted when attempting to reproduce a tachycardia previously documented to have occurred spontaneously.

Bradyarrhythmias

Sinus node dysfunction

Sinus node dysfunction is characterized by any of several types of rhythm disturbances, including sinus/junctional bradycardia, sinus pauses and episodes of supraventricular tachyarrhythmia (most commonly paroxysmal atrial fibrillation). Syncope can be caused by severe bradycardia (e.g., sinus pauses or sinus arrest), or may be associated with tachycardia. In the latter case, the faint may occur at the beginning of the paroxysm of atrial fibrillation (before blood vessels have had a chance to constrict adequately). Alternatively, it is not uncommon for syncope to be due to a long asystolic pause occurring at the end of an episode of atrial fibrillation (before the sinus pacemaker has an opportunity to resume at a relatively normal rate) (Fig. 14.7).

In patients with syncope of unknown origin, sinus node dysfunction can be suspected in the presence of severe sinus bradycardia (heart rates persistently < 50 beats/min), long asystolic pauses (Fig. 14.7) or episodes of sinoatrial block. The role of electrophysiologic testing for the diagnosis of sinus node dysfunction as a cause of syncope is limited. The tests used to evaluate the function of sinus node (sinus node recovery time and sinoatrial conduction time) exhibit good specificity, but they are relatively insensitive and may miss many affected individuals. Furthermore, with the possible exception of a very prolonged corrected sinus node recovery time (CSNRT), they do not provide direction regarding the appropriate treatment strategy for the patient.

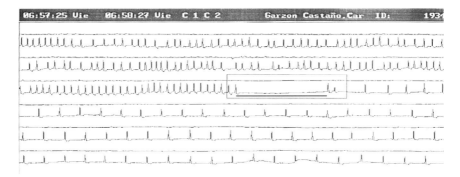

Fig. 14.7 Holter recording from a patient with syncopal episodes and sinus node dysfunction. Recording shows a period of atrial fibrillation with a rapid ventricular response that terminates abruptly. A 6-s asystolic pause was recorded before a regular rhythm resumes at approximately 50 beats/min.

The diagnosis of sinus node dysfunction leading to syncope is best established when a clear correlation of symptoms with arrhythmia (usually bradycardia) is documented. "Event" recorders or implanted loop recorders have the best chance of making the diagnosis by virtue of their long recording periods. In absence of such correlation, severe sinus bradycardia lower than 40 beats/min, repetitive sinoatrial block, or sinus pauses longer than 3 sec are highly suggestive of symptomatic sinus node disease.

In patients with sinus node dysfunction and syncope due to bradyarrhythmia, implantation of a pacemaker has been shown to improve symptoms. In these patients physiologic pacing (atrial or dual chamber) has been definitively shown to be superior to single chamber ventricular (VVI or VVIR) pacing. As these patients have an inappropriate chronotropic response, the use of rate-adaptive pacing is recommended.

In patients with paroxysmal atrial tachycardias associated with sinus node dysfunction, antiarrhythmic drug therapy may be needed. In such cases, however, aggravation of susceptibility to bradycardia may be unmasked. Once again, pacing may be a necessary element of therapy.

Atrioventricular conduction disorders

Chronic or paroxysmal atrioventricular (AV) block can be the cause of syncopal episodes. AV block may be congenital or an acquired disease.

Patients with congenital AV block can be severely symptomatic early in life or may remain asymptomatic for a long period of time. Previously, congenital AV block was considered a relatively benign condition. This is no longer the case. Follow-up studies have demonstrated that such patients, especially if they have suffered syncope, have an increased mortality. Consequently, it is now believed that they need to be treated aggressively with pacemakers.

Bradycardia due to intermittent AV block is among the more important causes of syncope. The presence of Mobitz II type 2nd degree AV block, 3rd degree AV block, or alternating left and right bundle branch block can be considered as diagnostic findings. In absence of these, there are other findings that can suggest that syncope may be due to AV block, but these additional findings are inferential only, and are not considered definitively diagnostic. Such observations include: presence of bifascicular block (left bundle branch block or right bundle branch block associated with left anterior or left posterior fascicular block); other intraventricular conduction abnormalities with a QRS duration longer than 120 ms; or documented Mobitz I 2nd degree AV block in older individuals. In the presence of these abnormalities further investigation should be performed to confirm the diagnosis, but the suspicion of AV block as the cause is important in directing the subsequent diagnostic plan.

In the evaluation of patients suspected of having paroxysmal AV block, conventional 24-h ambulatory ECG monitoring has low diagnostic yield since the chance of recording an event is low. An "event" recorder, and especially an implantable loop recorder (ILR), markedly extend the recording time and thereby improve the chance of detecting an abnormality (see Chapter 8).

ECG ambulatory monitoring can be considered diagnostic when a correlation between syncope and AV block is obtained. In the absence of such correlation, the presence of ventricular pauses longer than 3 sec when the patient is awake, or periods of Mobitz II or 3rd degree AV block can be considered diagnostic even in the absence of symptoms.

For patients with syncope of unknown origin and bifascicular block, or intraventricular conduction defects, an electrophysiologic study (EPS) is usually indicated. EPS in these patients should analyze not only the properties of conduction system, but also the inducibility of ventricular arrhythmias. The latter is particularly important in patients with structural heart disease. The assessment of the His–Purkinje system during EPS should include the measurement of baseline HV interval, incremental atrial pacing and, if baseline study is inconclusive, pharmacologic provocation with ajmaline, procainamide or disopyramide. An HV interval longer than 100 ms, the presence of 2nd or 3rd degree AV block with progressive atrial pacing, or high-degree A-V block after intravenous administration of ajmaline, disopyramide or procainamide, are considered sufficiently diagnostic findings. There is a difference of opinion regarding the significance of HV intervals of between 70 and 100 ms duration. In such cases, there may be suspicion that AV conduction disease is the source of the problem but it would be prudent to seek additional supportive information.

The absence of abnormal EPS findings in patients with syncopal episodes and bundle branch block does not exclude an arrhythmia as a possible etiology of syncope. In these patients implantation of a loop recorder (ILR, see Chapter 8) may be justified. Recent findings in the ISSUE trial strongly suggest that with prolonged recording periods (often 5–10 months is needed) it is ultimately possible to detect correlation between arrhythmia (often paroxysmal AV block) and syncope.

Tachyarrhythmias

Supraventricular tachyarrhythmias

Syncope is seldom due to supraventricular tachycardias. However, the recognition of these arrhythmias, and especially the paroxysmal supraventricular tachycardias (PSVTs), as a potential cause has importance as most of them can be successfully treated. More often, patients with supraventricular tachycardias experience palpitations. In those patients who develop syncope associated with supraventricular tachycardia, transient loss of consciousness usually appears at the beginning of the episodes before vascular compensation is possible. Some faints occur at the end of episodes, when an asystolic pause may occur before sinus rhythm resumes. In any case, the cause of syncope for patients with supraventricular tachycardias is usually multifactorial. Syncope is related not only to the increased heart rate, but also to an abnormal vasomotor response (i.e., delayed vasoconstriction) at the beginning of the arrhythmia that leads to more severe transient hypotension than would otherwise be expected. Susceptibility to syncope may also be increased in the presence of underlying sinus node disease. The latter predisposes to long post-tachycardia pauses at termination of the tachycardia.

PSVT due to AV nodal re-entry or accessory pathway

Except in those cases in which paroxysmal supraventricular tachycardia is documented in relation to syncopal episode, the recognition of an arrhythmic origin in these patients can be difficult. Most of these patients have no structural heart disease and, except in those patients with pre-excitation syndrome (e.g., Wolff–Parkinson–White syndrome), the baseline ECG is usually normal. Patients may recall palpitations, usually immediately before loss of consciousness; however, in many instances there is no recollection of unusual heart action. In those patients in whom PSVT is suspected, EPS is indicated. The induction of PSVT, especially if it provokes hypotension or reproduces clinical symptoms (this may not happen with the patient lying supine in the laboratory), can be considered diagnostic. More often than not, hypotension and symptom reproduction is only achieved if tachycardia is induced with the patient in an upright posture such as on a tilt-table. In any case, if tachycardia with a rapid rate consistent with the potential for hypotension is observed, radiofrequency catheter ablation is the treatment of choice.

Patients with evidence of pre-excitation on baseline ECG have additional clinical risks that may contribute to syncope (or even sudden death on rare occasion), and therefore need to be considered. In these patients, apart from paroxysmal AV re-entrant tachycardias, episodes of atrial fibrillation with very fast ventricular response (due to conduction over the accessory connection) can not only cause syncopal episodes but may also induce ventricular fibrillation leading to sudden death (Fig. 14.8). A similar example is also shown in Chapter 10. In these patients, radiofrequency catheter ablation is clearly the treatment of choice.

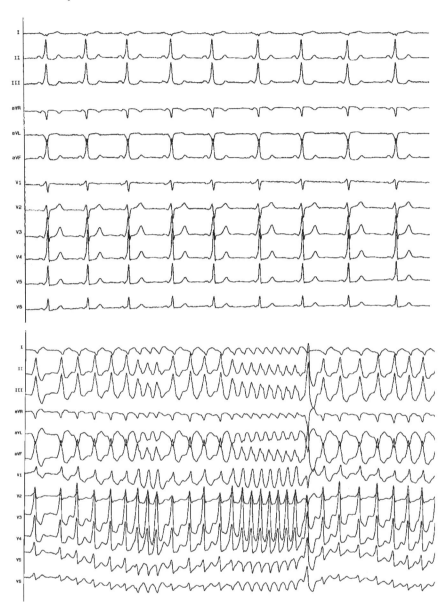

Fig. 14.8 ECG recording obtained from a patient with Wolff–Parkinson–White syndrome. The TOP trace is sinus rhythm with pre-excitation pattern suggesting a left lateral accessory connection. The BOTTOM panel shows a period of atrial fibrillation with a very fast ventricular response and varying degrees of pre-excitation. The rapid rate was associated with hemodynamic compromise sufficient to cause syncope.

Atrial fibrillation and atrial flutter

Patients susceptible to paroxysmal atrial fibrillation may also develop syncopal episodes. As noted earlier, syncope most often occurs at the beginning of the episode (before the vascular system has a chance to compensate by constricting). However, it may also occur at the end of the episode (especially in patients with concomitant sinus node dysfunction) when there may be a long asystolic pause before a regular heart rhythm resumes (Fig. 14.7).

It has also been shown that patients susceptible to syncope with paroxysmal atrial fibrillation often have an abnormal vasomotor response at the beginning of the arrhythmia. As discussed earlier, delayed vasoconstrictor compensation may play an important role in the the development of symptomatic hypotension. Finally, it is important to keep in mind certain special situations in which paroxysmal atrial fibrillation can cause acute hemodynamic deterioration leading to syncope. These high-risk situations include patients with advanced age, patients who are dehydrated or exposed to hot environments, and individuals with left ventricular outflow obstruction (e.g., hypertrophic cardiomyopathy, severe aortic stenosis).

Patients with atrial flutter have many of the same risks for syncope as do those with atrial fibrillation. However, two important additional considerations are important to bear in mind. First, exertion in patients with atrial flutter can lead to very rapid ventricular rates (e.g., 1 : 1 AV conduction). At such rapid rates, hypotension may ensue. Second, it has been reported that the use of class IC antiarrhythmic drugs in patients with atrial flutter, and even with atrial fibrillation, can slow the cycle length of the atrial tachyarrhythmia. Paradoxically, this slowing may reduce the degree of physiologic block offered by the AV node. The result is 1 : 1 AV conduction. Although the atrial rate may be "slower" than before the drug, the net ventricular rate is much faster due to 1 : 1 transmission. The result may be a sufficiently fast ventricular rate to cause severe hemodynamic compromise and syncope. When contemplating the use of antiarrhythmic drugs for treatment of atrial flutter (or similar atrial ectopic tachycardias) it is essential to try and avoid the risk of setting the stage for 1 : 1 AV conduction by concomitant administration of drugs that slow AV conduction, such as beta-blockers or calcium channel blockers. Alternatively, in the case of many forms of atrial flutter and atrial ectopic tachycardias, radiofrequency catheter ablation can eliminate susceptibility to the underlying arrhythmia, thereby avoiding the treatment problem entirely.

Ventricular tachycardias

Ventricular tachycardias (VTs) most often occur in patients with structural heart disease, especially ischemic heart disease and dilated cardiomyopathies. However, approximately 10–15% of patients that are diagnosed with VT have no structural heart disease. Ventricular tachycardias in patients without structural heart disease are often classified as idiopathic ventricular tachycardias.

Ventricular tachycardias associated with ischemic heart disease and dilated cardiomyopathies

Ventricular tachyarrhythmias have been reported to be responsible for syncope in up to 20% of patients referred for electrophysiologic assessment. Tachycardia rate, status of left ventricular function, and the efficiency of peripheral vascular constriction determine whether the arrhythmia will induce syncopal symptoms.

Non-sustained ventricular tachycardia is a common finding during ambulatory ECG monitoring, especially in patients with ischemic heart disease and dilated cardiomyopathies. Consequently, such a finding during the assessment of a syncope patient has not in the past been considered very helpful in the absence of documented concomitant symptoms. However, this view is changing, especially in patients with ischemic heart disease and severely diminished left ventricular function (i.e., ejection fractions < 35%), given the MUSTT and MADIT2 results. These studies suggest that such patients have a high mortality rate, and that implantable cardioverter defibrillator (ICD) therapy can be effective in diminishing mortality risk. Therefore, in the absence of other causes of syncope, the potential role of non-sustained ventricular tachycardia raises concern. In fact, based on the combined findings of MUSTT and MADIT2, it can be argued that ICD therapy may be warranted without undertaking an electrophysiologic study in ischemic heart disease patients with poor ejection fractions.

A persisting problem is the appropriate approach to be taken when syncope occurs in patients with severe underlying left ventricular dysfunction due to dilated cardiomyopathy. Consideration of prophylactic placement of an implantable cardioverter defibrillator (ICD) is becoming increasingly frequent in this setting, although the appropriateness of this strategy is uncertain. Completion of the SCD-HEFT study may shed some light on this dilemma. In the interim, the 2002 ACC/AHA/NASPE Guideline for pacemaker and antiarrhythmia device implantation provides a Class IIB indication for empirical ICD implantation in this setting irrespective of the etiology of the heart disease.

Idiopathic ventricular tachycardias and syncope

Right ventricular outflow tract tachycardia
Idiopathic right ventricular outflow tract (RVOFT) tachycardia is the most frequent type of idiopathic VT (Fig. 14.9). It represents approximately 80% of all idiopathic VT, and about 10% of all patients that are evaluated for VT. RVOFT tachycardia can be present at any age, but it is most frequently seen between the 2nd and 4th decade of life. It originates in the right ventricular outflow tract, and appears to be due to cyclic AMP-mediated "triggered activity". Typically RVOFT tachycardia can be terminated by adenosine administration, but this is of course only a temporizing step. The arrhythmia will recur if a more permanent solution is not provided (e.g., radiofrequency ablation).

RVOFT ventricular tachycardia is usually provoked by physical exercise. Patients with RVOFT tachycardia may be totally asymptomatic or they can experience palpitations, dizziness or syncope. Furthermore, although some

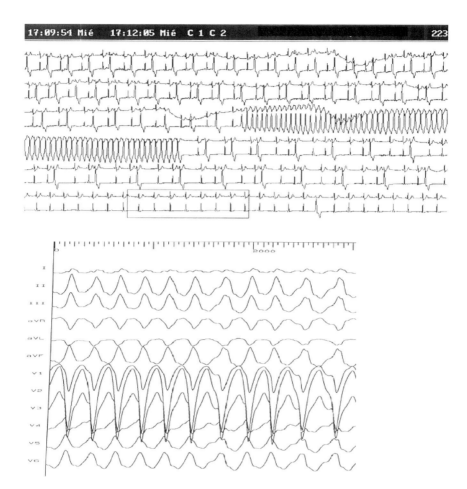

Fig. 14.9 Recordings obtained from a patient with sudden syncope, no apparent heart disease, and a normal ECG and echocardiogram. The TOP panel was obtained from a Holter recording showing sinus rhythm and frequent premature ventricular beats, followed by a rapid non-sustained ventricular tachycardia at 200 beats/min. The BOTTOM panel is a 12-lead ECG during isoproterenol infusion. The ventricular tachycardia has a left bundle branch block morphology suggestive of a right ventricular outflow tract origin. Radiofrequency ablation eliminated susceptibility to recurrent tachycardia.

sporadic cases of sudden death have been described, most often this tachycardia has a benign course from a mort-ality perspective. On the other hand, its associated symptoms may have a very negative impact on patient lifestyle.

Baseline ECG in these patients usually has a normal QRS. Some patients have frequent premature ventricular beats with the same morphology of tachycardia (i.e., a QRS which appears to have a left bundle branch block appearance but relatively narrow, with a vertical or rightward frontal axis)

(Fig. 14.9). Tachycardia in these patients can manifest as episodes of non-sustained VT, repetitive monomorphic VT interrupted by short periods of sinus rhythm, or episodes of paroxysmal sustained VT.

By definition, RVOFT tachycardia patients have no evident structural heart disease, but some minor abnormalities in the RV outflow tract have been described based on magnetic resonance imaging (MRI) techniques. As the morphology of this tachycardia can be similar to tachycardia observed in patients with a more worrisome condition called arrhythmogenic right ventricular dysplasia (ARVD), it is important that the second of these two conditions be excluded in each case.

In patients with syncope of unknown origin and no structural heart disease, ROVFT tachycardia should be suspected when syncopal episodes are associated with palpitations or when frequent premature beats or runs of non-sustained ventricular tachycardia with left bundle branch block and inferior (i.e., vertical or rightward) axis are seen at baseline ECG. Further diagnostic tests, such as repeated 24–48-h ambulatory monitoring or electrophysiologic study may be helpful in confirming the suspected diagnosis. During EPS the arrhythmia is typically induced during isoproterenol infusion with rapid atrial or ventricular pacing. Induction by programmed electrical stimulation alone is less reproducible.

Treatment is indicated in symptomatic patients with palpitations or syncope. Beta-blockers have been considered as the first-choice drug for the treatment of these patients. Other drugs that have been used effectively include calcium channel blockers, and class I and class III antiarrhythmic drugs. However, drug therapy has limited efficacy and possible side-effects. Furthermore, most of these patients are diagnosed at a relatively young age and are not optimal candidates for decades of drug treatment. Fortunately, radiofrequency catheter ablation of the arrhythmia site of origin has been used with a success rate of approximately 85%. Complications are uncommon, but include perforation of the RV wall leading to tamponade.

Idiopathic left ventricular outflow tract tachycardia

Idiopathic left ventricular outflow tract (LVOFT) tachycardia is less common than but analogous to RVOFT tachycardia. It exhibits subtle variations in QRS morphology during tachycardia, consisting mainly of the presence of an R wave in V1 and V2 leads. It has been shown, by intracavitary mapping techniques, that in these patients tachycardia originates at the left ventricular outflow tract (Fig. 14.10).

In these patients, as in patients with RVOFT tachycardia, syncope can be a clinical manifestation of the arrhythmia. In those cases, treatment with drugs may be considered, but radiofrequency catheter ablation is preferred.

Idiopathic left posterior fascicular tachycardia

This is the most frequent form of idiopathic left ventricular (LV) tachycardia. Although it can be present at any age, idiopathic LV fascicular tachycardia is

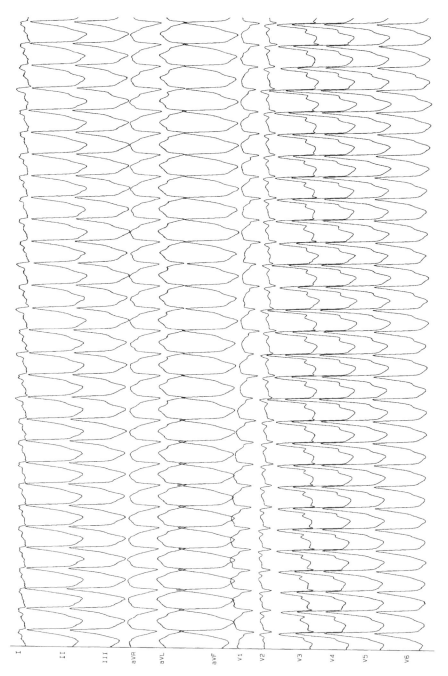

Fig. 14.10 Ventricular tachycardia in a patient without structural heart disease. The QRS has an inferior axis (i.e., positive QRS in inferior leads II, III, and aVF), and a left bundle branch block morphology, but with "r" waves from V2 suggesting an origin from the left ventricular outflow tract. Endocavitary mapping confirmed the activation site and radiofrequency ablation was successful.

most frequently seen in patients between the 2nd and 4th decade of life, and it predominates in males. The mechanism of tachycardia seems to be a re-entry in the left posterior fascicle. During EPS, the arrhythmia can usually be induced and stopped by programmed ventricular stimulation. Isoproterenol infusion does not facilitate induction, and the tachycardia is not affected by adenosine. Usually it can be easily terminated by verapamil infusion (although long-term oral verapamil is not generally effective for prevention of recurrences).

The most frequent form of presentation is as paroxysmal VT, with a QRS pattern of right bundle branch block and left axis deviation. Occasionally, similar right bundle branch block but with right axis deviation can be seen, suggesting that re-entry arises from the left anterior fascicle. Clinically, these patients may be asymptomatic, but when they have symptoms they usually experience palpitations, dizziness or syncope. Baseline ECG does not show specific abnormalities.

As in ROVFT tachycardia, the prognosis in these patients is generally benign, but some cases of sudden death have been reported. Consequently, symptomatic patients should be treated. Although this tachycardia responds to intravenous verapamil administration, chronic oral treatment is less effective, and in most of these patients radiofrequency catheter ablation can be performed safely and effectively.

Arrhythmogenic right ventricular dysplasia

Arrhythmogenic right ventricular dysplasia (ARVD) is a hereditary disease in which the right ventricular myocardium is replaced by fatty infiltration. The extent of infiltration can vary from minimal ventricular wall involvement, to a massive right ventricular replacement in the more severe forms of the disease. In some cases the left ventricle is affected as well.

The clinical picture ranges from asymptomatic patients to symptoms secondary to ventricular arrhythmias or right ventricular failure. In ARVD patients, ventricular arrhythmias are usually triggered by adrenergic stimulation. Syncope related to exercise should bring this diagnosis to mind.

Ventricular arrhythmias in ARVD patients can vary from isolated premature ventricular beats to non-sustained or sustained life-threatening VT. Clinical manifestations of ventricular arrhythmias in ARVD patients may vary from palpitations, to syncopal episodes, or even sudden death.

ARVD must be suspected in those patients with syncope of unknown origin with family history of premature sudden death or unexplained syncope, or when baseline ECG shows certain suggestive abnormalities. The most important of these abnormalities include: epsilon waves (a finding of a small late signal analogous to "late" potentials in ischemic heart disease, found in the ST segment, most often in V1 lead); low amplitude and localized prolongation of the QRS complex in leads V1 to V3; or inverted T waves in right precordial leads in the absence of right bundle branch block. In addition, some of these patients have frequent ventricular premature beats with a pattern of left bundle branch block suggesting a right ventricular site of origin.

Once suspected, the diagnosis of ARVD is best confirmed by specific imaging techniques, such as an echocardiogram, right ventricular angiography or MRI. These images can show dyskinetic areas, dilatation or depressed right ventricular function, and on occasion fatty replacement in the right ventricular wall. Moving image MRI (cine-MRI) is probably the best diagnostic tool currently available, but suffers from being expensive, not universally available, and perhaps overly sensitive. EPS can be helpful in inducing the ventricular arrhythmia and confirming the site(s) of origin.

An optimum treatment strategy for patients with ARVD and syncope has not been fully established. In some instances it has been suggested that antiarrhythmic drugs, specifically sotalol, and even radiofrequency catheter ablation can be effective. However, drug therapy is not well proven, and ablation success is limited by virtue of the potential for many regions of the heart to be affected and thereby become arrhythmogenic sites. Consequently, in those patients with syncope in which the presence of malignant ventricular arrhythmias can be demonstrated (either during a spontaneous recording or induced at EPS) an implantable cardioverter defibrillator (ICD) should be considered the safest treatment approach currently.

Long QT syndromes (primary, secondary)
The long QT syndromes may be a primary disorder or secondary to other factors (most commonly various drugs, Table 14.5). Drug-induced long QT syndromes are far more common than primary long QT, and new drugs capable of inducing the problem are being identified each year. The result is an increasing risk of iatrogenic syncope or even sudden death secondary to polymorphous ventricular tachycardia ("torsade de pointes"). Given the substantial public health hazard associated with drug-induced long QT, physicians must be very attentive to the risk. Eliminating the offending agent is the key to treatment.

The primary long QT syndromes comprise a group of disorders, generally familial in nature, and characterized by a prolongation of ventricular repolarization (i.e., long QT interval). These conditions predispose to "torsade de pointes" (Fig. 14.11). Syncope is one of the most common clinical presentations, but malignant ventricular arrhythmias can lead to sudden death.

Recently there has been considerable interest in the molecular biology of long QT syndromes and related conditions (e.g., Brugada syndrome, see later). The interested reader is referred to the growing comprehensive literature on this subject. It is only possible to provide a brief overview here.

Two main forms of "clinical" (phenotypic) presentation have been described for long QT syndrome. The most common is the so called Romano–Ward syndrome, which has an autosomal dominant pattern of transmission, and the second one is the so-called Jervell and Lange–Neilsen syndrome, which is inherited in an autosomal recessive pattern. Up to five different gene mutations have been identified for the Romano–Ward syndrome. These mutations appear to correlate with different patterns of clinical presentation.

Table 14.5 Drugs implicated in QT prolongation and torsades de pointes*.

Antiarrhythmic agents	*Psychoactive/antidepression agents*
Class IA	Phenothiazines
Quinidine	Thioridazine
Procainamide	Amitriptyline
Disopyramide	Imipramine
Class III	
Sotalol	*Antibiotics*
Ibutilide	Erythromycin
N-acetylprocainamide (NAPA)	Pentamidine
Dofetilide	Fluconazole
Amiodarone (relatively low risk)	
	Non-sedating antihistamines
Antianginal agents	Terfenadine (removed from market in USA)
Bepridil (removed from market in USA)	Astemizole
	Miscellaneous
	Cisapride (removed from market in USA)
	Arsenic
	Droperidol

*Only the more commonly used agents are listed here. A complete list is obtainable from the World Wide Web.

Although the most characteristic alteration at baseline ECG is an abnormal prolongation of QT interval, it has been recognized that there are some patients who have normal baseline QT interval duration. However, in many of these cases other abnormalities can be observed, such as T wave alternans or abnormalities in the morphology of T wave. These patients develop polymorphous ventricular tachycardias in the form of torsades de pointes that can degenerate to ventricular fibrillation. The arrhythmia is usually triggered by adrenergic stimuli.

Clinical manifestations may consist of syncopal episodes or sudden death. Syncope tends to begin at an early age, usually between 5 and 15. In the most common form of long QT syndrome syncopal episodes are usually triggered by adrenergic stimulus, such as exercise or stressful situations. However, other forms of long QT syndrome may result in torsades being triggered by bradycardia.

In patients with syncope of unknown origin, the presence of long QT syndrome must be suspected when there are abnormalities of repolarization, or family history of long QT syndrome, syncope or sudden death. There are several findings that when present seem to further enhance the risk of sudden death. These are: the presence of previous cardiac arrest; syncope at young age; family history of sudden death; a very prolonged corrected QT interval (QTc) (< 600 ms); and the presence of the recessive form of so called Jervell and Lange–Neilsen syndrome (i.e., long QT with hearing impairment).

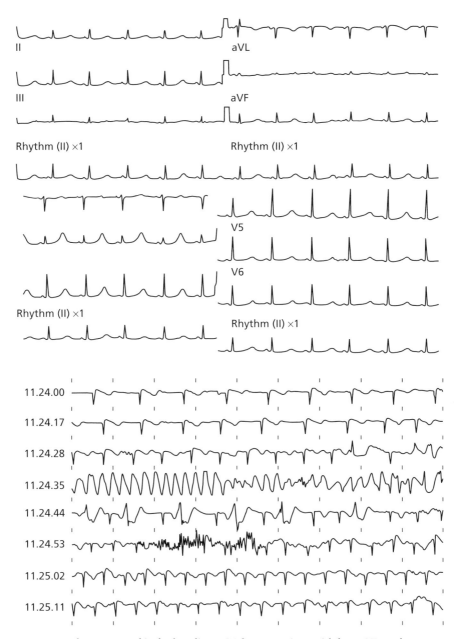

Fig. 14.11 The TOP panel is the baseline ECG from a patient with long QT syndrome and recurrent syncope. The faints were associated with triggers suggestive of a vasovagal etiology. The LOWER panel, obtained from an ILR placed subcutaneously in this patient, revealed a polymorphous ventricular tachycardia (torsade de pointes) to be the cause of a near-syncope event.

As a rule, patients with long QT syndrome should be advised to avoid vigorous exercise. They should also not be exposed to drugs that can further prolong QT interval (Table 14.5). For patients with a first syncopal episode and no other risk factors, treatment with beta-blockers is considered as a first-line treatment. When bradycardia-triggered syncope is implicated, the use of implanted cardiac pacemakers is justified. In patients that have other risk factors in addition to syncope (see above), or those who have syncope recurrences in spite of beta-blockers, implantation of an ICD is indicated. A strong family history of sudden death is probably a strong indicator for an ICD.

Brugada syndrome
In 1992, a group of eight patients who had experienced recurrent episodes of aborted sudden death without any apparent structural heart disease and in whom an distinct pattern at ECG was described. Further observations have resulted in this entity being recognized as an hereditary disease, characterized by an ECG pattern of right bundle branch block and ST elevation in V1 to V3. These individuals are at risk of developing episodes of polymorphous ventricular tachycardia. In addition it has been observed that the ECG can change over time in the same patient from a strictly normal ECG to the full characteristic pattern. In those patients with suspected Brugada syndrome who have an apparently normal ECG, intravenous administration of a Class I antiarrhythmic drug (e.g., procainamide) can provoke the typical QRS-ST segment changes, thereby confirming the diagnosis.

In patients with syncope of unknown origin the diagnosis of Brugada syndrome must be suspected when there is a family history of established Brugada syndrome, sudden death or unexplained syncope, or when baseline ECG shows the typical pattern. Although the risk of sudden death in asymptomatic patients with Brugada syndrome is not well known, it is now agreed that those patients who have had syncope or an aborted sudden death are at increased risk of sudden death. Currently available antiarrhythmic drugs are not useful in preventing arrhythmia recurrences in Brugada syndrome. Consequently, symptomatic patients or those with a strong family history of premature sudden death should be treated with an ICD.

Hypertrophic obstructive cardiomyopathy (HOCM)
Syncope may occur and be a presenting feature in conditions in which there is fixed or dynamic obstruction to left ventricular outflow such as valvular aortic stenosis or hypertrophic obstructive cardiomyopathy (HOCM). Symptoms are often provoked by physical exertion, but may also develop if an otherwise benign arrhythmia should occur (e.g., atrial fibrillation). Furthermore, even relatively slow ventricular tachycardias may cause syncope in such cases.

The basis for the faint is in part inadequate blood flow due to the mechanical obstruction. However, especially in the case of valvular aortic stenosis, ventricular mechanoreceptor-mediated bradycardia and vasodilatation is thought to be an important contributor. In obstructive cardiomyopathy, neural reflex mechanisms may also play a role, but occurrence of atrial tachyarrhythmias (particularly atrial fibrillation) or ventricular tachycardia (even at relatively modest rates) may trigger syncope.

Summary

Cardiac arrhythmias are important causes of syncope, particularly in patients with structural heart disease. Documentation of an arrhythmia in conjunction with syncope is the diagnostic gold standard for establishing the basis of symptoms. However, where this is not possible or clinically prudent, EPS may be warranted. However, EPS results may be misleading, and findings must be interpreted with care.

Further reading

Gann D, Tolentino A, Samet P. Electrophysiologic evaluation of elderly patients with sinus bradycardia: a long-term follow-up study. *Ann Intern Med* 1979; 90: 24–29.

Scheinman MM, Peters RW, Morady F, Sauve MJ, Malone P, Modin G. Electrophysiologic studies in patients with bundle branch block. *PACE* 1983; 6: 1157–1165.

Brignole M, Menozzi C, Moya A *et al.* Mechanism of syncope in patients with bundle branch block and negative electrophysiological test. *Circulation* 2001; 104: 2045–2050.

Leitch JW, Klein GJ, Yee R, Leather RA, Kim YH. Syncope associated with supraventricular tachycardia. An expression of tachycardia rate or vasomotor response? *Circulation* 1992; 85: 1064–1067.

Brignole M, Gianfranchi L, Menozzi C, Raviele A, Oddone D, Lolli G, Bottoni N. Role of autonomic reflexes in syncope associated with paroxysmal atrial fibrillation. *J Am Coll Cardiol* 1993; 22: 1123–1129.

Moss AJ, Schwartz PJ, Crampton RS *et al.* The long QT syndrome: prospective longitudinal study of 328 families. *Circulation* 1991; 84: 1136–1144.

Schwartz PJ *et al.* Stress and sudden death: the case of the long QT syndrome. *Circulation* 1991; 83(Supp II): 71–80.

Brugada J, Brugada P. Further characterization of the syndrome of right bundle branch block, ST segment elevation and sudden cardiac death. *J Cardiovasc Electrophysiol* 1997; 8: 325–331.

Knight BP, Goyal R, Pelosi F *et al.* Outcome of patients with non-ischemic dilated cardiomyopathy and unexplained syncope treated with an implantable defibrillator. *J Am Coll Cardiol* 1999; 33: 1964–1970.

Gregoratos G, Abrams J, Epstein AE *et al.* ACC/AHA/NASPE 2002 guideline update for implantation of cardiac pacemakers and antiarrhythmia devices: summary article. *Circulation* 2002; 106: 2145–2161.

Specific causes of syncope: their evaluation and treatment strategies

Part 4: Structural cardiac and pulmonary causes of syncope

Jean-Jacques Blanc, David G Benditt

Introduction

Structural cardiac, vascular or pulmonary diseases are uncommonly the direct cause of syncope. More often, the relationship of structural cardiopulmonary abnormalities to syncope events is indirect, by virtue of increased susceptibility to tachy- or bradyarrythmias, or hypotension of other cause (e.g., low cardiac output, acute myocardial infarction, etc.). In many of these cases a neural reflex mechanism contributes to the faint, e.g., syncope associated with acute myocardial ischemia, severe aortic stenosis or pulmonary hypertension. In any case, syncope associated with severe structural heart disease is a serious matter, and warrants immediate and thorough evaluation. Careful consideration needs to be given to hospitalizing these patients on an ECG-monitored cardiac station for their diagnostic evaluation, and often for initiation of therapy (especially if it entails use of antiarrhythmic medications).

Goals

The goals of this part of the chapter are to summarize:
- a scheme for risk stratification of syncope patients with structural cardiopulmonary disease; and
- the manner in which the diagnostic evaluation strategy differs from patients without underlying structural disease.

Risk stratification

Many different forms of structural cardiac and pulmonary disease may be associated with syncope. The most common are listed in Table 14.6. One study

Table 14.6 Common structural cardiac and pulmonary disease conditions associated with syncope.

Condition	Most common mechanism(s)
Acute myocardial infarction or ischemia	Reflex, reduced CO, VT
Chronic ischemic heart disease	VT, AV block
Aortic stenosis	Reflex
Atrial myxoma	Transient blood flow obstruction
Acute aortic dissection	Reflex
Pulmonary embolism	Reflex
Primary pulmonary hypertension	Reflex
Pericardial disease	Inflow obstruction, reduced CO
Dilated cardiomyopathy	VT
Arrhythmogenic right ventricular dysplasia	VT
HOCM	Outflow obstruction, VT

Abbreviations: CO, cardiac output; VT, ventricular tachycardia; AV, atrioventricular; Reflex, neural reflex vasodepressor/bradycardia; HOCM, hypertrophic obstructive cardiomyopathy.

has developed and validated a clinical prediction rule for risk stratification of patients with syncope. This study used a composite outcome of having cardiac arrhythmias as a cause of syncope or death (or cardiac death) within 1 year of follow-up. Four variables were identified and included age > 45 years, history of congestive heart failure, history of ventricular arrhythmias, and abnormal ECG (other than non-specific ST changes). Arrhythmias or death within 1 year occurred in 4–7% of patients without any of the risk factors and progressively increased to 58–80% in patients with three or more factors. The critical importance of identifying cardiac causes of syncope is that many of the arrhythmias and other cardiac diseases are now treatable with drugs and/or devices.

Most frequent causes

Structural cardiac or cardiopulmonary disease is often present in older syncope patients. However, in these cases it is more often the arrhythmias associated with structural disease that are the cause of syncope. In terms of syncope directly attributable to structural disease, probably the most common is that which occurs in conjunction with acute myocardial ischemia or infarction. Other relatively common acute medical conditions associated with syncope include pulmonary embolism and pericardial tamponade. The basis of syncope in these conditions is multifactorial, including both the hemodynamic impact of the specific lesion as well as neurally mediated reflex effects leading to inappropriate bradycardia and peripheral vascular dilatation. The latter is especially important in the setting of acute ischemic events, exemplified by the atropine-responsive bradycardia and hypotension often associated with inferior wall myocardial infarction.

Syncope is of considerable concern when it is associated with conditions in which there is fixed or dynamic obstruction to left ventricular outflow (e.g., aortic stenosis, hypertrophic obstructive cardiomyopathy, prosthetic valve malfunction). In such cases symptoms are often provoked by physical exertion, but may also develop if an otherwise benign arrhythmia should occur (e.g., atrial fibrillation). The basis for the faint is in part inadequate blood flow due to the mechanical obstruction. However, especially in the case of valvular aortic stenosis, neural reflex disturbance of vascular control is an important contributor to hypotension. In hypertrophic cardiomyopathy (HOCM), with or without left ventricle outflow obstruction, neural reflex mechanisms may also play a role. However, in HOCM, the occurrence of atrial tachyarrhythmias (particularly atrial fibrillation) or ventricular tachycardia (even at relatively modest rates) are important causes of syncopal events. Other less common causes of syncope in this class include left ventricular inflow obstruction in patients with mitral stenosis or atrial myxoma, right ventricular outflow obstruction, and right-to-left shunting secondary to pulmonic stenosis or pulmonary hypertension. The mechanism of the faint may once again be multifactorial, with hemodynamic, arrhythmic and neurally mediated origins in need of evaluation.

Vascular steal syndromes are very rarely the basis for syncope. Subclavian steal syndrome, albeit very uncommon, is perhaps the most important of these conditions and can reasonably be incorporated in the context of cardiopulmonary disease. Subclavian steal may occur on a congenital or acquired basis. Low pressure within the subclavian artery due to a stenosis in its most proximal portion near the aorta causes retrograde flow to occur in the ipsilateral vetebral artery (especially during upper arm exercise). The result is a diminution of cerebral blood flow. Syncope is typically associated with upper extremity exercise. Direct corrective angioplasty or surgery is usually feasible and effective. Other forms of vascular steal, particularly within the cranium, are recognized as potential causes of syncope, but are virtually impossible to diagnose.

Evaluation

Apart from identifying the nature and severity of any underlying cardiopulmonary disease in a patient with syncope, the cause of the faint needs special consideration. The same disease may induce syncope by different mechanisms. For example, acute myocardial infarction may initiate ventricular tachycardias or ventricular asystole (particularly in the case of inferior wall infarction). Similarly, faints during exertion in patients with severe valvular aortic stenosis can be due to inadequate cardiac output, or an inappropriate vascular response resulting in transient systemic hypotension. The latter is thought to be the more important. Syncope in patients with hypertrophic obstructive cardiomyopathy can also be the consequence of several mechanisms. Hypotension may again be due to direct obstruction to left ventricular ejection, but transient ventricular and atrial tachyarrhythmias as well as neural reflex causes are probably more common.

As has been emphasized throughout this volume, it is of major importance to consider whether structural cardiopulmonary disease is present in every patient with syncope. Two possibilities can be defined: cardiopulmonary disease is known to be present; or cardiopulmonary disease is not known to be present.

Cardiopulmonary disease is known to be present

In those cases where cardiopulmonary disease is known to be present and its severity is not thought to be critical, then only the mechanism of the syncope has to be determined. This aspect is readily solved if an arrhythmia has been registered during or immediately after the syncope episode. Conversely, and much more commonly, it is more difficult when there is no prior arrhythmia documentation. In such cases a complete hemodynamic assessment of the structural disturbance becomes essential, along with selection of appropriate tests to assess potential rhythm disturbances (see Chapters 8 & 10).

In cases where the presence of cardiopulmonary disease is known, but its severity has not previously been characterized, referral for selected non-invasive (e.g., echocardiogram, exercise testing, radionuclide imaging) and possibly invasive (e.g., angiography, hemodynamic measurements) evaluation is recommended. An arrhythmia or neural reflex event may have been the cause of the faint, but prognosis depends on the severity of the underlying disease.

Cardiopulmonary disease is not known to be present

When the structural cardiopulmonary disease is previously unknown two different circumstances need to be considered (Fig. 14.12). In an emergency setting (e.g., cardiogenic shock, acute severe prosthetic valve occlusion or regurgitation, acute chest pain) syncope is only one component of a complex clinical presentation. The presence of structural cardiopulmonary disease may now be obvious but its nature may be uncertain. Highest priority must be given to establishing the basis for acute decompensation and initiating appropriate treatment (e.g., acute pulmonary embolism, aortic dissection, myocardial infarction, papillary muscle or chordal rupture). In the second scenario, syncope is the only symptom, but ancillary factors such as patient age, medical history, family history and physical examination suggest the possibility of underlying structural cardiopulmonary disease. In such cases, it is reasonable to undertake straightforward low-risk non-invasive assessment to confirm (or set aside) the clinical suspicion. An ECG and echocardiogram are appropriate starting points. Depending on these findings, and physician comfort in assessing cardiovascular risk, referral for additional selected non-invasive (e.g., exercise testing, radionuclide imaging) and invasive (e.g., angiography, hemodynamic measurements) evaluation may be prudent.

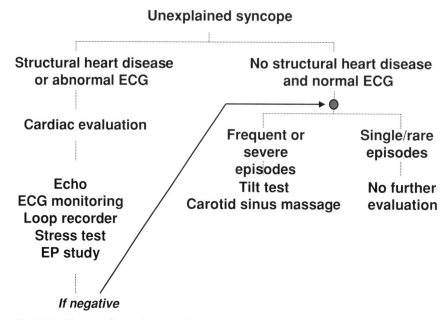

Fig. 14.12 Strategy for evaluation of patients with syncope who have structural cardiac or pulmonary disease.

Treatment

The treatment of syncope in the setting of structural cardiopulmonary disease is dependent on the nature and severity of the underlying structural abnormalities, and the apparent mechanism (i.e., arrhythmia, hemodynamic abnormality) leading to syncope. In an emergency situation the underlying structural disturbance must be treated first (e.g., acute myocardial infarction, severe aortic stenosis). Referral to a facility experienced in and capable of dealing with the problem is recommended. In non-emergency circumstances, treatment of the structural disease should be considered if feasible (e.g., aortic valve replacement in the case of severe aortic stenosis). However, in most cases it is reasonable to turn attention to determining the cause of syncope (e.g., ventricular tachycardia in dilated cardiomyopathy) and focusing on its treatment (e.g., antiarrhythmic drugs, ICD, etc.).

In syncope associated with acute myocardial ischemia, pharmacologic therapy and/or revascularization is clearly the appropriate strategy in most cases. Similarly, when syncope is closely associated with surgically addressable lesions (e.g., valvular aortic stenosis, atrial myxoma, congenital cardiac anomaly), a direct corrective approach is often feasible. On the other hand, when syncope is caused by certain difficult-to-treat conditions such as primary pulmonary hypertension or restrictive cardiomyopathy, it is often impossible to ameliorate the underlying problem adequately. There are no data on the effect of reducing outflow gradient on relief of syncopal relapses in HOCM.

It should be emphasized that for patients with structural cardiopulmonary disease, additional factors could participate in the triggering of a syncope event. For instance, electrolyte disturbances, increasing heart failure or worsening oxygenation may all facilitate arrhythmia initiation leading to syncope. Hypokalemia occurring as a side-effect of diuretic therapy is one of the most common scenarios to keep in mind. It is of course of crucial importance to recognize these triggering factors as their reversal can eliminate the symptoms.

Summary

Structural cardiac, vascular or pulmonary diseases are relatively uncommon causes of true syncope, but contribute to increasing susceptibility to faints by virtue of the increased risk of tachy- or bradyarrhythmias, or systemic hypotension of other causes. In any event, syncope associated with severe structural heart disease has a worrisome prognosis, and warrants immediate and thorough evaluation. Consideration needs to be given to hospitalizing these patients on an ECG-monitored cardiac station for their diagnostic evaluation, and often for initiation of therapy. As a rule, treatment is best directed at amelioration of the specific structural lesion or its consequences.

Further reading

Dixon MS, Thomas P, Sheridon DJ. Syncope as the presentation of unstable angina. *Int J Cardiol* 1988; 19: 125–129.

Johnson AM. Aortic stenosis, sudden death, and the left ventricular baroreceptors. *Br Heart J* 1971; 33: 1–5.

Nienaber CA, Hiller S, Spielmann RP, Geiger M, Kuck KH. Syncope in hypertrophic cardiomyopathy: multivariate analysis of prognostic determinants. *J Am Coll Cardiol* 1990; 15: 948–955.

Gosselin C, Walker PM. Subclavian steal syndrome. Existence, clinical features, diagnosis, management. *Semin Vasc Surg* 1996; 9: 93–97.

Specific causes of syncope: their evaluation and treatment strategies

Part 5: Cerebrovascular disorders as the primary cause of syncope

J Gert van Dijk

Introduction

As has been emphasized throughout this volume, neurologic disease is rarely the cause of true syncope. Neurologic disturbances may cause other forms of loss of consciousness, such as in the case of epilepsy. Similarly, traumatic neurologic disturbances may cause loss of consciousness by way of concussion. However, syncope (i.e., transient loss of consciousness due to inadequate cerebral perfusion) should not typically lead to a search for neurologic disease.

Goals

The goals of this part of the chapter are to:
- review the few important cerebrovascular conditions potentially associated with syncope; and
- emphasize the diagnostic differences between TIAs and true syncope.

Transient ischemic attacks (TIAs)

TIAs may resemble syncope in terms of being transient and self-limited. The similarity ends there, however. TIAs commonly last longer, and are associated with transient localizing neurologic signs and symptoms. The main difference lies in the symptomatology (Table 14.7).

Syncope basically concerns loss of consciousness without focal neurologic deficit; TIAs are the exact opposite: focal deficits without loss of consciousness. This holds without restrictions for carotid TIAs. Consequently, these two types of presentation do not cause any diagnostic confusion in neurology.

Table 14.7 Clinical findings: syncope versus carotid ischemia versus vertebrobasilar ischemia.

	Consciousness	Vision	Focal deficits
Syncope	Lost	May be impaired just before unconsciousness	None
Carotid TIA	Normal	Hemianopia or amaurosis fugax	*
Vertebrobasilar TIA	Rarely lost (not as isolated symptom)	Hemianopia	†

* Hemiparesis, hemianesthesia, aphasia, dysarthria, other higher cortical functions.

† Hemiataxia, diplopia, hemiparesis, dysarthria, vertigo, cranial nerve symptoms.

Vertebrobasilar TIAs are more likely to cause unconsciousness. However, once again, the symptomatology provides evidence for distinguishing this condition from true syncope. Vertebrobasilar TIAs are accompanied by focal deficits such as hemianopsia or ataxia, symptoms and signs which prove their nature as TIAs.

Subclavian steal

The subclavian steal syndrome may cause loss of consciousness, and can be detected by asking for circumstances provoking the attack. Physical exercise involving one arm suggests this entity, and should be followed by measuring blood pressure in both arms and ultrasound if necessary (see Chapters 12 & 14, Part 4).

Migraine

In individuals who suffer from migraine, syncope of an orthostatic nature occurs statistically more often than in non-migraineurs. These attacks do not occur at the same time as the migraine attacks, however, and so they can usually be distinguished without additional diagnostic confusion.

A rather rare type of vertebrobasilar migraine does involve impaired consciousness, but this lasts too long to cause confusion with true syncope. Nevertheless, making the diagnosis can be a challenge for most practitioners. Consequently, when migraine-related syncope is being considered, referral to a specialist experienced in these conditions is prudent.

Summary

Cerebrovascular disorders are only rarely the cause of syncope. Consequently, in the absence of focal neurologic signs or symptoms suggesting such a possibility, their evaluation should be considered a low priority. In essence, any testing directed toward cerebrovascular disease should be reserved for those instances in which the contribution of more likely potential causes of syncope have been excluded.

Further reading

Devuyst G, Bogousslavsky J, Meuli R, Moncayo J, de Freitas G, van Melle G. Stroke or transient ischemic attacks with basilar artery stenosis or occlusion: clinical patterns and outcome. *Arch Neurol* 2002; 59: 567–573.

Shechter A, Stewart WF, Silberstein SD, Lipton RB. Migraine and autonomic nervous system function. A population-based, case-control study. *Neurology* 2002; 58: 422–427.

CHAPTER 15

Syncope and other causes of transient loss of consciousness in children, teenagers and adolescents

Wouter Wieling, Karin S Ganzeboom, Jan Janousek

Introduction

Transient loss of consciousness is common in young subjects. It is a dramatic event not only for the patients involved, but also for other children, parents and teachers.

The main causes of transient loss of consciousness in the young are:
- syncope, a sudden transient fall systemic blood pressure resulting in a decrease in cerebral perfusion below a critical level necessary for mainten-ance of consciousness. Vasovagal syncope also called the common faint is by far the most common cause of transient loss of consciousness in young subjects;
- neurologic disorders, in particular epilepsy;
- psychiatric disorders mimicking true loss of consciousness, in particular conversion reactions (rare); and
- metabolic disorders (very rare).

Goals

The goals of this chapter are to review:
- epidemiology of syncope in children, teenagers and adolescents;
- initial approach to diagnosis;
- subsequent work-up; and
- therapy of syncope and certain other important causes of transient loss of consciousness.

Epidemiology

In children less than 6 years of age transient loss of consciousness is un-usual; breath-holding spells, cardiac arrhythmias and seizure disorders are the principal considerations when loss of consciousness does occur. This order of diagnostic consideration differs substantially from that recommended for older individuals.

In the general population a peak incidence of transient loss of consciousness is observed around the age of 15 years. The overall incidence of syncope coming to medical attention in childhood and adolescence is approximately 1 per 1000 (0.1%). By far the most common cause is a neurally mediated reflex syncopal disorder and in particular a vasovagal faint. The peak incidence of vasovagal fainting in the teenage period is thought to be related to the period of rapid growth. At the age of 20 years, about 20% of male subjects have experienced at least one vasovagal syncopal episode. The even higher prevalence in young women is thought to be related to the hormonal changes during the menstrual cycle. By comparison, in the general population in this same age group epilepsy has a prevalence of about 5 per 1000 (0.5%) and cardiac syncope (i.e., cardiac arrhythmias or structural heart disease) is even less common.

Initial approach to the diagnostic evaluation

A detailed patient and family history is the most crucial part of the initial diagnostic work-up of a young patient with transient loss of consciousness. The first challenge for the attending physician is to differentiate non-syncope conditions which cause apparent transient loss of consciousness (e.g., seizure disorders, drug intoxication) from true syncope (see Chapter 1 for definition). Then, the second challenge is to determine among the many young fainters whether a given patient falls within the small proportion of patients that are prone to serious and potentially lethal conditions such as arrhythmias and other cardiac causes of syncope and seizures. Most young fainters have more innocent causes of transient loss of consciousness, particularly neurally mediated reflex syncope.

The physical examination should focus on examination of the heart and measurement of blood pressure. Heart rate and blood pressure should be assessed with the patient both supine and after 3 min standing. A 12-lead surface electrocardiogram (ECG) is recommended to screen for rare forms of cardiac syncope, e.g., long QT syndrome, pre-excitation (e.g., Wolff–Parkinson–White syndrome), heart block (congenital or acquired) or ventricular hypertrophy.

Common causes of syncope in the young

Neurally mediated reflex syncope (neural reflex syncope)
Neurally mediated reflex syncopal disorders comprise a heterogeneous group of functional disturbances that are characterized by episodic reflex vasodilatation and/or bradycardia resulting in transient failure of blood pressure control (Fig. 15.1). The pathophysiologic and clinical aspects of these disorders are dealt with in Chapters 2 and 14, Part 1, respectively.

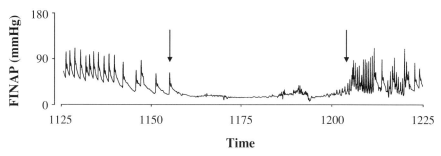

Fig. 15.1 Blood pressure recording obtained in a 17-year-old boy with frequent faints due to blood injury phobia when a blood taking provocation was discussed. Just mentioning the procedure induced 50 sec of asystole. (Finapres recordings.) Arrows: 1, last heartbeat before asystole; 2, first heartbeat after asystole, coinciding with the start of resuscitation. Time (s) taken from the original registration. (From N van Dijk *et al. PACE* 2001; 24: 122–124 with permission of the editor.)

Reflex syncopal disorders have an excellent prognosis, but may have serious social repercussions and a dramatic impact on the quality of life. Diagnosing these disorders is therefore of great importance. In most young patients without heart disease, if the history is typical, and the physical examination and ECG is normal, then a presumptive diagnosis of reflex syncope can be made without any other testing. Many young subjects with reflex syncope have a history of syncope in an immediate family member which has not been associated with sudden death and this may be helpful in formulating the differential diagnosis.

The main triggers causing neural reflex syncope in the young are similar to those in older people, and are listed in Table 15.1. The more common specific neurally mediated faints are described below.

Vasovagal syncope
In young subjects vasovagal syncope is the most common of the neural reflex disorders (Fig. 15.1). Two situations in particular are known to provoke this disorder. First, distressing emotional situations and pain can induce a vasovagal faint. The pathways involved descend from the corticohypothalamic centres in the brain to medullary cardiovascular centres. A typical example is an ordinary faint during blood drawing (Fig. 15.1). This condition is more common in young subjects than in adult subjects. Emotional triggers for vasovagal syncope or near-syncope in children and teenagers include having a hair cut, eye examinations, placing a contact lens, dental procedures, or watching television programs about medical matters or animal biology.

Factors that increase pooling of venous blood below the heart such as long periods of standing motionless in combination with high ambient temperatures are also known to precipitate vasovagal syncope.

Young subjects often experience prodromal symptoms and signs when a spontaneous vasovagal syncope is imminent (Table 15.2). These prodromal symptoms are reported to be more intense than those in elderly subjects,

Table 15.1 Triggers of neurally mediated reflex faints in the young.

Emotional circumstances and pain, venipunctures, immunizations

Prolonged motionless standing, especially in combination with warm temperature, confined
    spaces, crowded rooms ("church syncope")

Fasting, lack of sleep, fatigue, menstruation, illness with fever

Micturition

(Post)exercise (i.e., after termination of long runs or vigorous bursts of activity during
    competitive sports)

Hyperventilation and straining (self-induced syncope)

Stretching

Coughing

Standing up quickly or arising from squatting

Pronounced weight loss

Certain medications, alcohol and drugs (these need to be distinguished from intoxicated
    states which can also cause loss of consciousness)

Table 15.2 Typical premonitory
symptoms for vasovagal faints in
young subjects.

Lightheadedness
Palpitations
Weakness
Dimming or blurred vision
Nausea, epigastric distress
Feeling warm or cold
Facial pallor
Sweating, dilated pupils

perhaps related to a more intact cerebrovascular supply and a more robust
autonomic nervous system responsiveness, and there is less complete disrup-
tion of memory during a vasovagal episode in the young. However, some
young subjects have little or no prodromal symptoms, and the collapse occurs
without warning of any kind.

In young subjects with recurrent episodes of apparent vasovagal reflex syncope the presentation can vary markedly, encompassing the classical emotionally induced vasovagal episodes, posture-induced vasovagal syncope, and
occasional vasovagal episodes with no consistent trigger. Apparently benign
vasovagal episodes may even occur during normal daily exercises like playing,
walking or cycling. Thus, the clinical presentation may vary widely both
within and among young patients.

Other forms of neurally mediated reflex syncope

Situational faints are common in young patients. In this regard the description
of these conditions is similar to that provided in Chapter 14, Part 1 for older

patients. Carotid sinus syndrome, on the other hand, is not a consideration in young patients (except in the rare case of a child who may have been subjected to neck surgery and/or radiation therapy to the neck).

Orthostatic syncope: postural orthostatic tachycardia syndrome (POTS) and autonomic failure

An orthostatic disorder that has received much attention lately is the so-called postural orthostatic tachycardia syndrome (POTS). It is defined by symptoms of cerebral hypoperfusion (e.g., lightheadedness, fatigue, weakness, blurred vision) and an excessive increase in heart rate in the upright posture (postural tachycardia). Other symptoms of sympathetic activation such as diaphoresis, nausea and tremulousness may also occur.

Postural tachycardia is related to age, with lower values in older age groups. Thus the normal ranges need to be adjusted for age. We consider an increase in heart rate of > 35 beats/min or to > 120 beats/min in upright posture as excessive. The female : male ratio of the postural orthostatic tachycardia syndrome is about 4–5 : 1. Fainting occurs in a minority of the subjects. The underlying mechanisms are debated. Partial denervation of the lower limbs as well as central nervous system functional disorders have been suggested as the basis for this disorder. When it is severe in terms of impact on well-being and lifestyle, POTS patients require evaluation at a specialty center in order for the diagnosis to be confirmed and treatment recommended. Mild forms of POTS are reasonably treated in the community. The prevalence in the general population is not known, but is probably low.

Primary autonomic neuropathy as a cause of orthostatic hypotension and syncope is extremely rare in young subjects. Secondary autonomic neuropathy with symptomatic orthostatic hypotension and (near-)syncope may occur in the setting of chronic diseases like diabetes mellitus and in young patients using vasoactive medications.

Additional distinctive syncopal syndromes observed in the young

Fainting lark

Non-reflex-mediated factors that are involved in fainting in young subjects include hyperventilation, where the decrease in Pa_{CO_2} causes constriction of cerebral vessels. Straining which impedes venous return may also trigger syncope. These adjunctive factors, in conjunction with prolonged orthostatic stress, have been reported to be involved in epidemic syncope in female teenage fans during rock concerts. They are also incorporated in self-induced fainting. The latter stunt has been used by children, high school students and military recruits as entertainment for their friends, and by others for more practical purposes such as avoiding imminent exams. The "fainting lark" is the maneuver most commonly used. It combines the effects of acute arterial

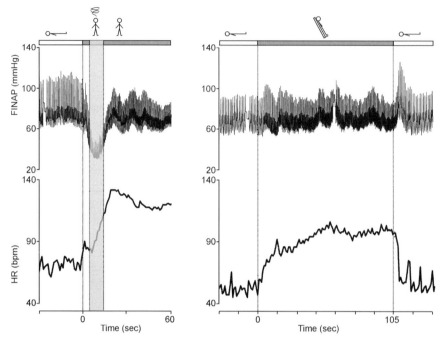

Fig. 15.2 Changes in heart rate and blood pressure in a 20-year-old male with an asthenic habitus (197 cm and 73 kg) and a 10-year long history of almost daily near-syncope and occasional syncope upon standing up. Note the marked initial fall in finger blood pressure accompanied by lightheadedness upon active standing, but not upon a passive head-up tilt. (Revised from N van Dijk *et al. Ned Tijdschr Geneesk* 2000; 144: 249–254 with permission of the editor.)

hypotension induced by standing up quickly, and raised intrathoracic pressure with cerebral vasoconstriction due to hypocapnia. The "fainting lark" is initiated by the subject first squatting in a full knee bend and then overbreathing. The subject then stands up suddenly and performs a forced expiration against a closed glottis. Almost instantaneous syncope with little or no warning symptoms occurs. The fainting lark has also been applied as a research tool to study the sequence of events during fainting in young adults (for more details see Chapter 2).

Syncope upon standing up

Syncope or near-syncope upon standing is another relatively distinctive syncopal syndrome observed in young subjects (although similar symptoms also occur in older individuals) (Fig. 15.2). Almost all young subjects are familiar with a brief feeling of lightheadedness shortly after standing up quickly, characterized by its time of onset (5–10 sec after standing up) and short duration (disappearance of symptoms within 30 sec). The complaints occur especially after prolonged supine rest or after arising from the squatted position. In some instances true syncope may occur upon standing in otherwise healthy teenagers and adolescents. The complaints are caused by a transient fall in systemic blood pressure, which occurs upon active standing, but not so dramatically (or not at all) upon passive head-up tilt (Fig. 15.1). The initial transient fall in blood pressure in healthy subjects is ascribed to vasodilatation in the active muscles during standing up. The majority of the patients involved are reported to be tall with an asthenic habitus and poorly developed musculature.

Stretch syncope

Stretch syncope may occur during stretching with the neck hyperextended while standing. It is reported to occur in teenage boys with a familial tendency to faint. It has been attributed to effects of straining (which decreases systemic blood pressure) in combination with decreased cerebral blood flow caused by mechanical compression of the vertebral arteries. The latter element of the pathophysiology seems somewhat unlikely, but cannot be excluded.

Migraine

Migraine-related syncope is another syncopal syndrome thought to occur predominantly in young subjects. It has been reported with prodromal symptoms that suggest brainstem ischemia due to basilar artery involvement (brainstem migraine). A typical attack starts with bilateral visual symptoms, dysarthria, rotational vertigo, diplopia, nystagmus, ataxia and transient loss of consciousness, followed by a headache that is usually bioccipital and throbbing. The headache may not always be present. Patients are often adolescent females with a positive family history. Other symptoms and signs of vasomotor dysregulation, in particular Raynaud's phenomenon, are often present. A role for orthostatic syncope in migraine sufferers has also been reported (see Chapter 14, Part 5).

Breath-holding spells

Between the age of 0 and 4 years the most common cause of syncope is what has been termed breath-holding spells, but they are only occasionally triggered by true breath-holding. In many cases there is a familial history. There are two types of breath-holding spells.

- Pallid breath-holding spells occur if there is a sudden fright, a fall or slight trauma. The crying phase is short or absent and often described as a "silent cry" mimicking a Valsalva maneuver. The loss of consciousness occurs within seconds and is associated with hypotonia, which passes into rigidity with myoclonic jerks. Marked pallor is observed. The condition is most commonly caused by a vagally mediated cardiac inhibition.
- Cyanotic breath-holding spells are usually elicited by unpleasant emotionally charged situations. They usually happen if the child is upset or angry. Crying occurs at the beginning which increases in intensity and finally terminates with prolonged expiration and visible cyanosis. Loss of consciousness and hypotonia followed by a few myoclonic jerks often occur. The

etiology of cyanotic breath-holding spells is not entirely clear. However, a few scenarios have been hypothesized including hypocapnic cerebral vasoconstriction due to hyperventilation during the crying phase, cerebral hypoxia due to hypoventilation and reflex closure of the vocal cords inducing a Valsalva-like increase in intrathoracic pressure and intrapulmonary shunting with ventilation–perfusion mismatch. Importantly, syncope in toddlers may also occur unassociated with any event or crying, but is often still labeled as a "breath-holding" spell.

Less frequent causes of syncope in the young

Cardiac syncope

Cardiac etiology should be considered first in patients who have any of the following:
- congenital or structural heart disease (including postoperative congenital heart disease, long QT syndrome, obstructive cardiomyopathy);
- few, if any, prodromal symptoms suggestive of neurally mediated reflex syncope;
- palpitations or chest pain as prodrome;
- syncope induced by exercise, auditory stimuli, swimming or diving; or
- a positive family history for unexplained cardiac syncope or sudden death.

Arrhythmias

Arrhythmias tend to be the most common cause of cardiac syncope in young subjects. Table 15.3 summarizes the conditions of greatest concern predisposing to arrhythmic causes of syncope. Myocardial dysfunction is seldom a direct cause of syncope in young subjects. Exceptions are certain individuals with a cardiomyopathic picture resulting from congenital heart disease or on an idiopathic basis. In such cases susceptibility to symptomatic arrhythmias is increased.

The syncope that occurs in the congenital long QT syndromes is due to the hemodynamic compromise caused by a polymorphous "torsade de pointes" ventricular tachycardia (Fig. 15.3). Most patients exhibit their first event in the first two decades of life. Episodes have been associated with fright, being awakened by a loud noise or extreme emotional stress. Other triggering causes include diving and exercise. In many patients there is a positive family history of sudden death. The various forms of long QT syndromes (LQTS) and related "ion channelopathies" have been the subject of intensive study in recent years. The reader is referred to detailed reviews of the subject.

Ventricular tachycardia (VT) due to right ventricular dysplasia may be associated with syncope, often associated with exercise. However, sustained and non-sustained symptomatic VT can occur at any time.

In patients with Wolff–Parkinson–White (WPW) syndrome and other forms of ventricular pre-excitation, either paroxysmal supraventricular tachycardia

Table 15.3 Most important conditions associated with arrhythmias in the young.

Tachycardias

Postoperative congenital heart disease (e.g., ventricular septal defect repair, tetralogy of
  Fallot)

Hypertrophic obstructive cardiomyopathy (HOCM)

Pre-excitation syndromes, especially Wolff–Parkinson–White syndrome and concealed
  accessory AV connections (common)

Long QT syndrome (rare but potentially life-threatening ventricular tachyarrhytmias,
  torsades)

Brugada syndrome (rare, but life-threatening ventricular tachyarrhythmias)

Arrhythmogenic right ventricular dysplasia (relatively common, but variable manifestations)

Idiopathic ventricular fibrillation (rare)

Bradycardias

Acquired atrioventricular block (relatively rare, but occurs more frequently with
  postoperative congenital heart repairs)

Congenital AV block (syncope is now known to be more common than previously thought)

Acquired sinus node dysfunction (again most often seen with postoperative congenital heart
  repairs)

Familial sinus node disease (rare)

Bradycardia–tachycardia syndrome

Atrial or ventricular arrhythmias after surgical treatment for congenital heart disease
  (common)

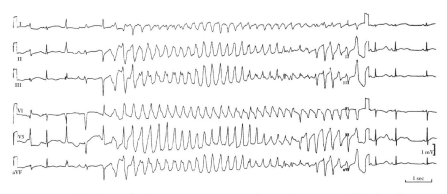

Fig. 15.3 Six-lead ECG (leads I, II, III, AVF, V1 and V5) of a 14-year-old girl with
syncopal attacks typically triggered by auditory stimuli. The tracings show a 10-s
episode of torsades de pointes, which terminate spontaneously. Grossly abnormal
QT intervals are observed immediately after termination of the arrhythmia. Long
QT syndrome (LQTS) type 2 was diagnosed. (Courtesy of AAM Wilde, Professor of
Experimental Cardiology, Academic Medical Center, Amsterdam, The Netherlands.)

alone or atrial fibrillation with a rapid ventricular response can be the cause of syncope. Many young patients may have paroxysmal supraventricular tachycardia using concealed accessory pathways and exhibit no evidence of pre-excitation. The re-entry mechanism is identical to that of conventional WPW narrow QRS tachycardia, and both are curable with catheter ablation techniques.

With a hypotensive tachycardia or marked bradycadia the patient may appear to be pulseless and may have myoclonic jerks and urinary incontinence. Recovery is typically rapid with a sudden return of the pulse, flushing of the face and usually full orientation of the patient. Certain of these rhythm disturbances may, however, lead to life-threatening consequences.

Primary obstructive cardiac causes of syncope

Obstructive conditions causing syncope in the young are in many respects similar to those seen in older subjects, with the exception of atherosclerotic cardiovascular disease which is rarely encountered in young individuals. As is true in older subjects, the basis of the faint may be the hemodynamic limitation imposed by the lesion, but could also be the result of arrhythmias or even neural reflex events. Multiple causes of syncope need to be kept in mind when contemplating therapy strategy. Obstructive conditions of particular importance in young subjects are:

* valvular/supravalvular aortic stenosis;
* hypertrophic cardiomyopathy (HOCM);
* primary pulmonary hypertension;
* tetralogy of Fallot;
* postoperative congenital heart disease (especially ventricular septal defect repair); and
* Eisenmenger's syndrome.

Psychogenic causes ("pseudo-syncope")

A conversion reaction is a rare cause of apparent transient loss of consciousness in young subjects. However, it may occur in adolescents, and predominantly in females. Consideration should be given to this diagnosis in the instance of a relatively high frequency of syncope recurrences (up to several times a day), and absence of associated physical injury. The duration of the loss of consciousness is often prolonged. During an episode tightly closed eyes or voluntary lid closure with lid flutter can be observed, while during true syncope or epilepsy the eyes are often open and deviated. An unusual posture may be assumed. Some of these patients are found to have suffered from sexual abuse or battering. Malingering with simulated convulsions (pseudo-seizures) has also been reported in young subjects as a cause of transient loss of consciousness. Finally, illicit substance abuse, in particular of alcohol and cocaine, is associated with exotic unexplained episodes of syncope in young subjects. The reader is referred to Chapter 13 for additional discussion of psychogenic "pseudo-syncope".

Table 15.4 Distinguishing myoclonic jerks from the abnormal motor activity associated with "grand mal" (generalized) seizures.

In neurally mediated reflex syncope, myoclonic jerks start after the subject has fallen on the floor, whereas in epilepsy the tonic clonic movements start while standing

Young subjects having an ordinary faint normally become very pale, while patients having a seizure may be cyanotic

In epilepsy the duration of the loss of consciousness is longer (usually > 5 min), whereas in reflex syncope loss of consciousness is usually short (often 1 min or less)

Urinary incontinence can happen both in reflex syncope and in epilepsy but seems to be more common in epilepsy

Loss of bowel control suggests epilepsy

Tongue biting almost exclusively occurs in epilepsy

Postictal confusion always happens in epilepsy and is prolonged, whereas it is less intense and shortlasting in reflex syncope. However, prolonged fatigue may occur after reflex syncope and is very characteristic of the vasovagal faint

The ability to stand upright occurs in epilepsy before complete recovery of mental function, whereas in reflex syncope it usually occurs after complete recovery of mental function (although the patient may remain "fatigued")

Distinguishing syncope and epilepsy

Myoclonic jerks mimicking a seizure may occur during vasovagal syncope and in other forms of syncope as well. An asystole of about 10 sec duration is needed in adults before myoclonic jerks occur. In young persons the anoxic threshold is reported to be lower than in adults. It is lowest in early childhood. Clinical features known to be helpful for distinguishing myoclonic jerks from the abnormal motor activity associated with "grand mal" seizures are summarized in Table 15.4.

Subsequent diagnostic work-up

The history and the physical examination guide the attending physicians in choosing the subsequent diagnostic work-up. In the case of a history typical for reflex-mediated syncope (e.g., vasovagal faint, postmicturition syncope, etc.), the absence of abnormalities on physical examination and a normal ECG are usually sufficient to make a diagnosis. Further investigations are not necessary. The work-up for other than reflex-mediated syncopes is case specific.

Ambulatory ECG (AECG) recorders should be used for patients with a history of palpitations associated with syncope. Whether to choose a 24-h, 48-h or longer-term recorder depends on the anticipated frequency of attacks suggested in the medical history. Implantable loop recorders (ILRs) may be parti-cularly effective in cases of troublesome but infrequent syncope. Cardiology consultation including echocardiography should be obtained in the case of a heart murmur. Whenever syncope occurs during exertion or emotion an echocardiogram and an exercise test should be performed in addition to the careful history, physical examination and ECG. Electro-encephalography (EEG) is indicated for patients showing prolonged loss of consciousness, seizure activity and a significant postictal phase of lethargy and confusion. The EEG is not, however, recommended as a "screening tool" in the evaluation of fainters.

Electrophysiologic study has a very minor role in pediatric patients with syncope, especially in the absence of structural heart disease. Testing may be warranted if a tachyarrhythmia is suspected, particularly in the case of operated congenital heart disease, HOCM, arrhythmogenic right ventricular dysplasia (ARVD), and pre-excitation syndromes.

In patients with "atypical" vasovagal syncopes or unexplained syncope and a normal cardiac evaluation, tilt-table testing can be helpful. Such testing may not be warranted given a single syncope, but is warranted if a second occurrence develops and in patients with multiple faints. Head-up tilt tests may have a relatively high "false-positive" rate (15–20% in adults) and should therefore be used with caution for the primary identification of patients with vasovagal syncope. The false-positive rate may be higher in children and adolescents than in adult patients, especially after instrumentation (e.g., placement of venous or arterial cannula): an incidence of near-fainting of 40% was reported during a head-up tilt test after placement of a simple intravenous line in healthy children and teenagers. The false-negative rate in adults has been estimated to be as high as 50%, but this number is uncertain as many of these "false negatives" subsequently have faints (suggesting that the test may have identified a susceptible individual). In young subjects the "false-negative" rate is probably lower.

Tilt-table testing can be helpful for patients with conversion reactions. In such cases loss of consciousness may occur with little or no significant decrease in heart rate, blood pressure or cerebral blood flow. A normal EEG may be observed during monitored episodes. Further, the patient can be observed by the physician, and typical markers of vasovagal syndrome are absent.

Therapy

The cause of the syncopal event determines the appropriate therapy. Therapy for other than reflex-mediated syncopes like cardiac arrhythmias and seizures is straightforward and case specific. Since vasovagal syncope is so common in this age group, it is reasonable to discuss its treatment strategy in greater detail.

Aborting the acute episode

For acute management of the vasovagal faint (and certain situational faints), recognition of warning symptoms and subsequent resumption of the supine position is usually sufficient. Elevation of the legs may be performed in order

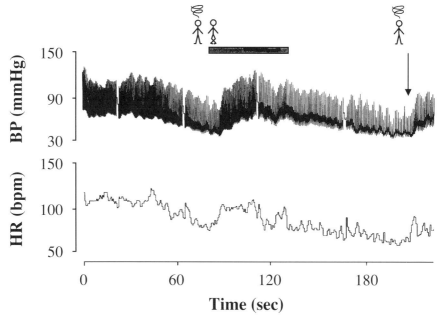

Fig. 15.4 Aborting a vasovagal faint by the combination of leg crossing and muscle tensing. In a 15-year-old female subject with recurrent syncope, a typical vasovagal syncope episode was induced during orthostatic stress testing on a tilt-table. Note progressive fall in finger arterial pressure and heart rate. After crossing of the legs and tensing of leg and abdominal muscles blood pressure and heart rate recover quickly. After uncrossing of the legs a vasovagal reaction is observed (arrow), and the subject has to be returned to supine position. Bar indicates onset of leg crossing and muscle tensing. (From Krediet and Wieling, unpublished.)

to increase venous return to the heart. Traditionally sitting with lowering the head between the knees has been advocated to abort an attack.

Instruction to apply physical countermaneuvers that can decrease downward pooling of venous blood and thereby increase stroke volume and cardiac output at the earliest recognition of presyncope is helpful in many young patients. We have found the combination of leg crossing and muscle tensing easily taught and effective in young patients with reflex syncope (Fig. 15.4) (see also Chapter 2). Patients are advised to use leg crossing as a preventive measure to improve orthostatic tolerance under stressful conditions and to combine leg crossing with tensing of leg and abdominal muscles when a faint is imminent (Fig. 15.4). Squatting can be used as an emergency measure to prevent loss of consciousness when presyncopal symptoms develop rapidly. A major advantage of applying physical countermaneuvers is that they can be applied immediately at the start of hypotensive symptoms, and the patient can regain self-confidence in stressful situations.

Long-term treatment options

In the long term, the most important point in patients with neural reflex syncope is explanation (education) and reassurance regarding the nature of the condition. Patients should be informed that there is minimal risk of sudden death, but that physical injury is still of some concern. Initial advice should include early recognition of warning symptoms and avoidance of triggering events. A tilt-table test can be employed for explanation and to teach the patient to recognize early premonitory symptoms in a safe setting. The frequency of syncopal events decreases substantially after tilt-table testing. It has been suggested that the clinical encounter, education and counseling that are associated with this diagnostic procedure have the effect of a positive therapeutic intervention.

A low salt diet should be avoided. Advice for "superhydration", i.e., enough liquid intake to produce colorless urine at a frequency of twice in the morning and twice in the afternoon may help. Two glasses of water with meals is a practical advice. During sporting activities and when symptomatic, "electrolyte" (NaCl)-containing liquids, which expand the extracellular fluid volume, should be advised. These may also be used on routine days to facilitate hydration.

In highly motivated patients with recurrent vasovagal symptoms, the prescription of progressively prolonged periods of enforced upright posture (so-called "tilt training") is reported to reduce syncope recurrence. The mechanism underlying its effectiveness is unknown. Compliance with this procedure limits its use in our experience in young subjects.

In young patients with vasovagal reflex syncope due to blood phobia, psychologic deconditioning is the first choice of therapy. In one to five sessions, dependant on the seriousness of the phobia, patients are exposed to phobic stimuli and taught to apply body tension. Prognosis after psychologic counseling seems to be very good.

Pharmacologic therapy should be reserved for the rare patient with continued symptoms despite behavior modification. However, undesirable side-effects associated with the drugs often outweigh any proposed effects. Additionally, pharmacologic treatment is less successful for hypotension induced by physical exercise or in warm surroundings. Another unresolved issue is for how long prophylactic therapy with any compound should be advised, since reflex syncope is a self-limited, non-life-threatening condition. Beta-blockers are often used, but the overall evidence in their favor is weak. Despite the absence of controlled studies, the mineralocorticoid fludrocortisone is often used early in the management of vasovagal syncope in an attempt to increase blood volume in young subjects. The combination with increased salt intake is required for an optimal effect. Fluid retention and hypertension in young subjects are reported to be less problematic than in the elderly. Other medications include alpha-adrenergic agonists like midodrine or pseudoephedrine to increase the peripheral vascular resistance and venous tone.

Even in the instance of cardioinhibitory syncope with an exaggerated asystolic response, pacemaker therapy should be avoided whenever possible.

Effective management with conventional therapy without the need for pacemaker implantation is almost always effective and clearly preferable in young patients. It seems sensible to reserve pacing for young subjects who have repeatedly exhibited prolonged asystole during a typical attack. In most cases an implantable loop recorder needs to be implanted to document such episodes. Breath-holding spells generally do not require specific therapy unless connected with long asystole periods associated with potential cerebral injury.

Summary

Syncope is common in children, teenagers and adolescents. It is usually attributable to neurally mediated reflex syncope, but the differential diagnosis includes other less common, but potentially dangerous disorders such as cardiac dysrythmias or ventricular outflow tract obstruction. The most important part of the diagnostic evaluation is taking a good history. An ECG is a helpful screening tool for the rare cardiac causes. The patient's symptoms before and after the syncopal episode and an observer's description of the event will help to determine the cause in the vast majority of patients. If there is doubt about the diagnosis, cardiac causes must be ruled out and ultimately a tilt-table test can be done. The mainstay of management of young patients with reflex syncope consists of advice and education on the various factors that influence systemic blood pressure in conjunction with chronic expansion of the intravascular volume or reducing the vascular volume into which pooling occurs.

Further reading

Saul JP. Syncope: etiology, management, and when to refer. *J South Carolina Med Assoc* 1999; 95(10): 385–387.

Driscoll DJ, Jacobsen SJ, Porter CJ, Wollan PC. Syncope in children and adolescents. *J Am Coll Cardiol* 1997; 29(5): 1039–1045.

Tanaka H, Yamaguchi H, Matushima R, Tamai H. Instantaneous orthostatic hypotension in children and adolescents: a new entity of orthostatic intolerance. *Pediatr Res* 1999; 46(6): 691–696.

Van Dijk N, Velzeboer SCJM, Destree-Vonk A, Linzer M, Wieling W. Psychological treatment of malignant vasovagal syncope due to blood phobia. *PACE* 2001; 24: 122–1224.

Krediet CTP, Van Dijk N, Linzer M, Van Lieshout JJ, Wieling W. Management of vasovagal syncope: controlling or aborting faints by the combination of leg crossing and muscle tensing. *Circulation* 2002; 106: 1684–1689.

Low PA, Sandroni P, Singer W, Benrud-Larsen L, Novak V, Schondorf R. Postural tachycardia syndrome—an update. *Clin Autonom Res* 2002; 107–109.

Priori SG, Barhanin J, Hauer RNW *et al.* Genetic and molecular basis of cardiac arrhythmias: impact on clinical management. Parts I and II. *Circulation* 1999; 99: 518–528.

CHAPTER 16

Syncope in the older adult (including driving implications)

David G Benditt, Rose Anne Kenny

Introduction

Syncope in older individuals presents several important unique problems. First, older patients are more likely to be unable to provide a detailed medical history due in part to a greater tendency to retrograde amnesia for premonitory events, and in some cases failing mental capacity. Second, unlike younger generally healthy patients, the elderly fainter is more likely to have multiple coexisting medical issues, any one of which could account for a faint, thereby complicating the evaluation due to the potential for multiple causes of syncope to be present. Third, the older frail individual is at higher risk for significant physical injury, especially bony fractures and subdural hematomas. Finally, susceptibility to faints in the elderly is more likely to result in loss of an independent lifestyle, and lead to being prematurely institutionalized. The latter two issues are of particular importance given the enormous cost burden of health care in old age.

Goals

The objectives of this chapter are to:
- highlight certain unique features associated with the evaluation of transient loss of consciousness in the older individual; and
- provide insight into diagnostic concerns which tend to be more important in the elderly.

Causes of syncope in the elderly

The commonest causes of syncope in older adults are orthostatic hypotension (often drug-induced), neurally mediated syncope (particularly carotid sinus hypersensitivity) and cardiac arrhythmias.

Orthostatic hypotension (see also Chapter 14, Part 2)

The prevalence of orthostatic hypotension in older adults varies from 6% in community-dwelling elderly, to 33% in elderly hospital inpatients. Orthostatic hypotension is an attributable cause of syncope in 20–30% of older patients. In symptomatic patients up to 25% have "age-related" orthostatic hypotension, in the remainder orthostatic hypotension is predominantly due to medications, primary autonomic failure, secondary autonomic failure (diabetes) and Parkinson's disease. Supine systolic hypertension is often present in older patients with orthostatic hypotension. Hypertension may increase the risk of cerebral ischemia from sudden declines in blood pressure, but it also complicates treatment, given that most agents used for the treatment of orthostatic hypotension will exacerbate supine hypertension.

Neurally mediated reflex syncope

Neurally mediated reflex syncope is relatively frequent in older individuals; however, unlike in younger patients, prescription drug-related triggers and carotid sinus hypersensitivity are far more prevalent in the older fainter. Over half the episodes are related to prescription of cardiovascular medications. The pattern of blood pressure and heart rate responses during testing is similar to that described in younger patients (see Chapter 9), although patterns reflecting dysautonomia are common.

Carotid sinus hypersensitivity is an age-related diagnosis. It is rare before the age of 50 years, and the prevalence increases with advancing years and with cardiovascular, cerebrovascular and neurodegenerative comorbidity. Cardioinhibitory carotid sinus syndrome has been considered in recent reports to be an attributable cause of symptoms in up to 20% of faints, but further study is needed. Nevertheless, carotid sinus syndrome is more common than was previously thought.

Up to 20% of syncope in older patients is due to cardiac arrhythmias. The reader is referred to Chapter 14, Part 3 for more details. In brief, though, older patients with syncope and bundle branch block are now thought to have a relatively high predilection to transient symptomatic high-grade atrioventricular (AV) block, and many of them will ultimately prove to need cardiac pacemakers.

Diagnostic evaluation

In the elderly patient, an initial evaluation comprising a detailed history, clinical examination, orthostatic blood pressure measurement and supine and upright carotid sinus massage will provide a diagnosis in over 50% (see Chapter 5). However, about one third of elderly patients will have more than one possible attributable cause for syncope. Consequently, it is important to be open-minded in undertaking the assessment, and utilize selected tests to confirm suspected diagnoses when there is any doubt.

History-taking

Aspects of history-taking in older adults may vary in emphasis and clinical details from younger adults. This is explained in some by amnesia for loss of consciousness. Gait and balance instability and slow protective reflexes are present in 20–50% of community-dwelling elderly. In these circumstances moderate hemodynamic changes insufficient to cause syncope may result in falls. Therefore, it is important to obtain an eye-witness account of episodes, although this may not be possible in many instances. Up to one third of syncope events will present as "falls", meaning that the patient will not recall having lost consciousness but does recollect being on the ground.

Cognitive impairment is present in 5% of 65 year olds and 20% of 80 year olds. Cognitive status will influence the accuracy of recall for events. The history should include details of social circumstances, injurious events, impact of events on patient confidence and sense of being able to remain independent in terms of carrying out activities of daily living without help.

The time when events occur can be also be helpful for diagnosis. Events due to orthostatic hypotension usually occur in the morning. The history should include any association with meals (postprandial), ingestion of medications, nocturnal micturition, etc. One third of over 65 year olds are taking three or more prescribed medications. Medications frequently cause or contribute to syncope. Details of the medication history should include duration of treatment and time relationship of this to the onset of events.

The history should include details of comorbid diagnoses, in particular associations with physical frailty and locomotor disability (e.g., arthritis, Parkinson's disease and cerebrovascular disease) and diagnoses which increase the likelihood of cardiovascular syncope (e.g., diabetes, anemia, hypertension, ischemic heart disease and heart failure).

Physical examination

Elderly patients have a high prevalence of cardiac disease. Consequently the careful cardiac and peripheral vascular examination may pay handsome dividends in older syncope patients. Evaluation for extra heart sounds and murmurs may suggest the presence of significant structural heart disease. An echocardiogram is then usually warranted to provide quantitative assessment. On the other hand, carotid bruits, although relatively frequent in this population, are almost never the cause of the problem. The physician should not be overly aggressive with neurologic tests in such cases, unless evident neurologic signs are present, or the history is more suggestive of a seizure than syncope.

Assessment of the neurologic and locomotor systems, including observation of gait and standing balance (eyes open, eyes closed), is recommended as part of the initial evaluation in older patients. However, in most cases a basic assessment can be adequately provided by the emergency department physician or the general practitioner. On the other hand, if cognitive impairment is suspected, this should be formally evaluated. The mini mental state examination is a 20-item, internationally validated tool, adequate for this purpose. Otherwise the clinical examination is as for younger adults.

Investigations

In cognitively normal older patients with syncope or unexplained falls the diagnostic work-up is largely the same as for younger adults. Exceptions include routine supine and upright carotid sinus massage, given the high prevalence of carotid sinus syndrome as a cause of syncope and unexplained falls in the older age group. In up to a third of older patients a diagnostic cardioinhibitory (i.e., demonstration of an induced pause of > 5 sec duration) response is only present when upright; reasons for this are unclear but may relate to technique or changes in reflex sensitivity with postural change.

Orthostatic hypotension is not always reproducible in older adults. This is particularly so for medication-related or age-related orthostatic hypotension. Repeated morning measurements are recommended. Twenty-four-hour ambulatory blood pressure recordings may be helpful if medication-induced or postprandial hypotension is suspected. However, the methodology of obtaining ambulatory blood pressure recordings is a limiting factor. Current techniques (e.g., repetitive sphygmomanometer measurements) may interfere with the autonomic changes that the physician is trying to record. In older patients with orthostatic hypotension, diurnal patterns of blood pressure are the mirror image of normal blood pressure behavior, being highest at night and lowest in the mornings (and possibly after meals). Knowledge of diurnal blood pressure behavior can guide treatment, and may be particularly helpful in modifying the timing of medications.

If symptoms continue or more than one diagnosis is suspected further evaluation is necessary. There is no evidence to support the use of head-up tilt studies as part of the initial evaluation, although this is common practice in many facilities. Otherwise, the same criteria as for evaluation of younger adults apply.

Evaluation of the frail elderly

Age *per se* is not a contraindication to assessment and intervention. However, in frailer patients, the rigor of the assessment will depend on compliance with tests, overall prognosis, and of course patient and family wishes. Orthostatic blood pressure measurements, carotid sinus massage and head-up tilt studies are well tolerated tests, even in the frail elderly with cognitive impairment. If patients have difficulty standing unaided, head-up tilt can be used to assess orthostatic blood pressure changes. If invasive diagnostic procedures and repeated hospital admissions are deemed inappropriate it may be necessary to treat "blind" using limited clinical data, i.e., by altering possible culprit medication, prescribing antiarrhythmic agents and/or cardiac pacing. Thus, in the frail elderly, physicians should make clinical judgements, after a comprehensive examination, about the benefits to the individual of a syncope evaluation.

There is some evidence that modification of cardiovascular risk factors for falls/syncope reduces the incidence of subsequent events in community-dwelling frail elderly, even those with dementia, but there is as yet no evidence of benefit for institutionalized elderly. Whether or not treatment of hypotension or arrhythmias decelerates cognitive decline in patients with dementia is not known.

Driving and syncope

Most medical causes of road accidents occur in drivers who are already known to have pre-existing disease. Thus older drivers are more likely to be at risk in terms of syncope, and also perhaps sleep disorders. Younger drivers tend to be more susceptible to driving impairment as a consequence of various forms of intoxication or lack of attention.

Sudden driver incapacity has been reported with an incidence approximating only 1/1000 of all traffic accidents. Apart from intoxicated states such as occur with alcohol or other drugs, the medical condition of a driver tends not to be an important factor in road accidents causing injury to others. The most common causes of road accidents involving presumed syncope at the wheel are listed in Table 16.1.

In an American Heart Association (AHA)/North American Society of Pacing and Electrophysiology (NASPE) medical/scientific statement dealing with personal and public safety issues related to arrhythmias that may affect consciousness, proposed recommendations on driving after syncope. Recommendations were provided for the following groups of drivers and the reader is referred to that publication for details.

- Drivers of ordinary motor cycles, cars and other small vehicles with and without a trailer.
- Drivers of vehicles over 5 metric tonnes or passenger-carrying vehicles exceeding 8 seats excluding the driver.
- Drivers of taxis, small ambulances and other vehicles which form an intermediate category between the ordinary private driver and the vocational driver.

Table 16.1 Causes of 2000 road accidents involving collapse at wheel, based on reports by the police to Driver Vehicle Licensing Agency.

Epilepsy	38%
Blackouts	21%
Diabetes on insulin	18%
Heart condition	8%
Stroke	7%
Others	7%

The present guidelines listed aim at being practical and enforceable. The guidelines reflect a combination of clinical judgement and some individual technical measurements. For ordinary drivers the task force advises minimal restrictions and thus only temporarily should patients with heart disease and syncope in this group be advised not to drive. However, local government regulations should be consulted before making a final recommendation. Professional drivers may need prolonged restriction (6 months or longer) until an effective treatment is demonstrated.

Summary

The evaluation of mobile, independent, cognitively normal older adults is as for younger individuals. However, risk factor stratification, and the contribution of individual abnormalities to symptom reproduction are more complex than in healthier younger individuals. Multiple risk factors are more common in the elderly and the boundaries between falls and syncope are poorly delineated. Patients have a median of five risk factors for syncope or falls. As a rule though, morning orthostatic blood pressure measurements and supine and upright carotid sinus massage are integral to the initial evaluation unless contraindicated. In frailer older adults evaluation should be modified according to prognosis. Driving and avocation restrictions must consider local government regulations, and should be individualized.

Further reading

Lipsitz LA, Wei JY, Rowe JW. Syncope in an elderly, institutionalized population: prevalence, incidence, and associated risk. *Q J Med* 1985; 55: 45–54.

Wollner L, McCarthy ST, Soper NDW, Macy DJ. Failure of cerebral autoregulation as a cause of brain dysfunction in the elderly. *Br Med J* 1979; 1: 1117–1118.

Jansen R, Penterman BJM, Van Lier HJT, Hoefnagels WHL. Blood pressure reduction after oral glucose loading and its relation to age, blood pressure and insulin. *Am J Cardiol* 1982; 60: 1087–1091.

Shannon RP, Wei JY, Rosa RM *et al*. The effect of age and sodium depletion on cardio-vascular response to orthostasis. *Hypertension* 1986; 8: 438–443.

Lipsitz LA, Nyquist P, Wei JY, Rowe JW. Postprandial reduction in blood pressure in the elderly. *N Engl J Med* 1983; 309: 81–83.

Scheinberg P, Blackburn I, Rich M *et al*. Effects of aging on cerebral circulation and metabolism. *Arch Neurol Psych* 1953; 70: 77–85.

Herner B, Smedby B, Ysander L. Sudden illness as a cause of motorvehicle accidents. *Br J Int Med* 1966; 23: 37–41.

Driving and heart disease. Task Force Report. Prepared on behalf of the ESC Task Force by MC Petch. *Eur Heart J* 1998; 19: 1165–1177.

Epstein AE, Miles WM, Benditt DG, Camm AJ *et al*. Personal and public safety issues related to arrhythmias that may affect consciousness: implications for regulation and physician recommendations. *Circulation* 1996; 94: 1147–1166.

CHAPTER 17

Conditions that mimic syncope

J Gert van Dijk

Introduction

Certain medical conditions may cause a real or apparent loss of consciousness which might appear to be syncope, but which is in fact not a true syncope. In order to understand which conditions may mimic syncope, we must take one step upwards on a hierarchical tree of definitions towards a larger entity—transient loss of consciousness—of which syncope is a subset.

Syncope is defined as a transient, self-limited loss of consciousness, with a rapid onset, spontaneous and prompt recovery, and *caused by global cerebral hypoperfusion.* That final element of the definition is crucial to understanding not just what syncope is, but also what the differential diagnosis may be. In essence, "syncope mimics" are conditions that are also associated with "transient loss of consciousness" or seem to be associated with "transient loss of consciousness", but are not the result of cerebral hypoperfusion.

Since there are so many different possible causes of transient loss of consciousness, it is important to have an overview of the various causes of transient loss of consciousness. With this background, practitioners can consider each presentation carefully, beginning with a detailed medical history; without it, physicians may resort to a wasteful "shotgun diagnostic approach", ordering tests for all disorders that may possibly cause transient loss of consciousness (or even testing for some that do not).

Goals

The goals of this chapter are to:
- provide a framework for syncope as part of the larger group of conditions causing "transient loss of consciousness";
- discuss non-syncopal disorders with real transient loss of consciousness;
- discuss disorders with apparent transient loss of consciousness; and
- provide help with disentangling the clues.

A framework

Most physicians will think of consciousness as "a degree of alertness". In this concept, unconsciousness is a total loss of alertness, i.e., something resembling sleep but from which one cannot be awakened. Consciousness resides either in the brainstem or in the integrity of a very large part of the cerebral cortex. The best syncope mimics may therefore be found among disorders affecting the function of these structures. Epilepsy is the foremost of these.

There is also a wider concept of consciousness, including not just the degree of alertness but also its nature. This may seem vague, but trances, hypnosis or even daydreaming affect the awareness of oneself or the surroundings, and also affect responsiveness. In other words, consciousness can be altered instead of just lost. This type of disorder may also mimic syncope, but is less impressive than conditions that cause total loss of alertness.

"Transient loss of consciousness", if taken at face value, may result from many disorders including concussion of the brain, hypoglycemia, intoxication, subarachnoid hemorrhages, and others that do not really resemble syncope that much; there are too many differences in clinical presentation. Disorders that do mimic syncope obviously have transient loss of consciousness (TLOC) in common, but several other features as well.

- A short duration, of usually not more than a few minutes (coma does not belong in the same list as syncope).
- TLOC must be self-limited (conditions requiring resuscitation do not usually cause confusion with syncope).
- TLOC should not be due to external trauma to the head. (This is mainly to exclude a concussion, which can easily be differentiated from the other causes of TLOC in the vast majority of cases, which are all caused by some internal process in the patient rather than due to an external cause.)

Bearing these points in mind, we may define "TLOC" as a *transient, short-lived and self-limited loss of consciousness not due to an external cause*. By its very nature, this means that doctors usually do not see patients during TLOC, but only afterwards. Most clues to select the precise cause of TLOC in a given patient will therefore have to be unearthed through careful history-taking.

In some cases the basis for syncope may be readily apparent. For instance, TLOC in a nervous young girl immediately following ear piercing: this is almost certainly a case of reflex syncope. Note that while an external factor plays a part here, it is only a *trigger*; the *cause* of the unconsciousness is cerebral hypoperfusion, which is of an internal rather than external nature (see Chapters 2 & 14, Part 1). Another example is a TLOC accompanied by first unilateral and then generalized jerking movements in a known epileptic: this should be considered an epileptic seizure, unless there are overwhelming arguments for something else. Then again, what does one do with someone who had a "spell" or "attack" in a busy shopping center, in whom "some jerks" were reported, but for whom otherwise no eye-witness account is available? Epilepsy? Syncope? In some cases, it may not even be possible to establish that

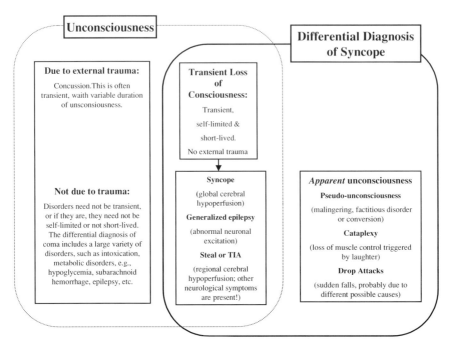

Fig. 17.1 Syncope and associated disorders were ordered according to clinical presentation. Assuming unconsciousness, "transient loss of consciousness" (TLOC) is defined by four other elements. Syncope belongs in this group. Altering one or more of the four items of TLOC results in a presentation for which one must consider other disorders in which unconsciousness occurs. No attempt was made to divide this group in subsets. Other disorders in which unconsciousness is only seemingly lost, but which otherwise have a similar clinical presentation, are bundled under "apparent unconsciousness". Together with the TLOC group these constitute disorders in the differential diagnosis of syncope.

consciousness was indeed lost; all that is clear is that there was an attack of some sort in which consciousness *looked* lost.

This chapter will not only deal with non-syncopal disorders causing TLOC, but will also go into disorders in which consciousness is only apparently lost (Fig. 17.1). However, before doing so, we may consider which entities are encountered by changing some of the items in the list of criteria that define TLOC; altering any one of them changes the list of possible disorders. How about an elderly woman, living alone, who has a bump on the head and little recollection of events? The bump might be due to a syncope-related fall, or the unconsciousness might also have been the result of head trauma caused by stumbling. If we cannot be certain whether the head trauma was the cause rather than the result of unconsciousness, we have to consider TLOC as well as a concussion. Another series of disorders come into play when the items "short-lived" or "transient" are altered. In that case, metabolic disorders, intoxication and other neurologic disorders, including structural cerebral damage, will have to be considered. Fig. 17.1 shows the results of these mental exercises.

Real, non-syncopal transient loss of consciousness

Epilepsy

Epilepsy is, like syncope, clinically characterized by (usually) transient (usually) short-lived attacks of a (usually) self-limited nature. For some, the word "seizure"is limited to epileptic attacks, while for others it may denote attacks from other causes as well. Here, the word "seizure" will be used as a synonym for "epileptic attack". From this point on, there may be two important differences from syncope. The first is that the pathophysiology is totally different, and the second is that consciousness need not be lost.

Epilepsy is due to aberrant functioning of neural networks. Somehow they escape their normal firing pattern. The result is uncontrolled firing of cortical neurons. What this does to the patient is simply the result of which functions are governed by the misbehaving neurons. Thus, any cortical function may appear as a result of epilepsy. Hence, seizures may take the form of simple movements, but sensations affecting any sense, emotions, thoughts and complex behavior patterns may also be due to epilepsy. The brain area that functions abnormally often changes in the course of an attack, and this is reflected in a changing clinical expression. For instance, the textbook aura, in which the patient experiences a strange sensation welling upwards from the abdomen, or senses a strange smell or unprovoked fear, signifies that only a small portion of the cortex is actually out of control. If the abnormal activity spreads to motor areas, movements may be seen which, depending on the spread of abnormal activity over the cortex, may first affect one limb or body side, or affect all limbs simultaneously. The international classification of epilepsy (Table 17.1) is based on the concept of spreading activity: the two main categories are partial seizures, beginning locally in a part of the cortex, and generalized ones, without an apparent local beginning.

Epilepsy and consciousness

As epilepsy is a disorder of the cerebral cortex, it is logical that generalized forms of epilepsy, affecting the cortex bilaterally, cause unconsciousness (Table 17.1). This is the form of unconsciousness with a total loss of alertness; the other type, in which consciousness is altered, also occurs in epilepsy; in fact, partial seizures are divided according to whether or not consciousness is "impaired". The best-known examples of this type are complex partial seizures in adults and absence epilepsy in children (true absence epilepsy is very rare in adults). In complex partial seizures, patients may first stop what they are doing and stare. Later, they may sit, walk, look around, perform inappropriate

Table 17.1 Classification of epilepsy (shortened). Forms of epilepsy that are relevant in the differential diagnosis of syncope are noted by an asterisk (*).

---

1 *Partial seizures (seizures beginning locally)*
  A Simple partial seizures (consciousness not impaired)
    Attacks may be motor, sensory, psychic or autonomic in nature
  B Complex partial seizures (with impairment of consciousness)
    In such cases consciousness may be altered at the start of the attack, but this may also develop during it
  C Partial seizures with secondary generalization

2 *Generalized seizures (bilaterally symmetric and without local onset)*
  A Absence seizures
  B Myoclonic seizures
  C Clonic seizures*
  D Tonic seizures*
  E Tonic–clonic seizures*
  F Atonic seizures*

3 *Unclassified epileptic seizures* (This category is used when there are inadequate or incomplete data to use the other two groups)

---

actions, such as relocating objects, and even vaguely and inappropriately answer questions. Such attacks may last from seconds to many minutes. During absences, children often freeze their actions, but will stay upright. They will stare or blink repeatedly, not respond to being spoken to, and may have "automatisms", such as chewing or lip movements. Attacks of these types do not really resemble syncope. There is probably little chance of them being mistaken for epilepsy, or the other way around. They may resemble the situation that may be seen in subjects with orthostatic hypotension before actual syncope. In such cases cerebral hypoperfusion may for a while be low enough to impair consciousness without causing its complete loss.

Types of epilepsy that may mimic syncope

Returning to differential diagnosis, there are five forms of epilepsy (Table 17.1) to consider for the present purpose. These are subdivided according to the type of movement.

"Myoclonic" refers to bilateral jerks, alone or in short series, usually without impairment of consciousness; this type needs not concern us. "Tonic" here refers to the body and limbs being held in a stiff position, usually with the limbs extended. "Clonic" refers to coarse, large-scale and powerful jerking movements of the arms and legs. These are usually synchronized over the body. "Tonic–clonic" refers to a succession of stiffness and movements. During the tonic phase the patient may utter a cry and may keel over like a falling log. Thereafter massive synchronous jerking movements occur. These gradually decrease in frequency and severity. This scenario lasts for a period of varying length, but usually only about a minute (estimates of bystanders are usually much longer than the actual duration). Finally, "atonic" seizures, as the name suggests, are not accompanied by movements of any kind. Nevertheless, control over postural muscles is lost. Patients fall limply to the floor, with flaccid muscles. Such attacks often last only long enough to cause a fall, and then it may not be clear whether consciousness was lost. Attacks may however, last for 1 min or longer, and are then accompanied by unconsciousness. Luckily for differential diagnosis, atonic attacks are rare, and almost exclusively seen in small children.

Short-listing Table 17.1 leaves four types of epilepsy that may be mistaken for syncope or vice versa. It should be understood that both stiffness and jerking movements may definitely occur in syncope. Both have been observed in intentionally provoked syncope (using the so-called "mess trick"). Most subjects fell limply, but a minority fell rather stiffly to the floor in a manner resembling epilepsy. Jerking movements occurred in no less than 90% of cases; this observation is extremely important, as both lay people and most medical and paramedical personnel commonly assume that jerking movements equal epilepsy. Luckily, the movements differed from those seen in epilepsy: in syncope, the movements were smaller, and not synchronous over various parts of the body. The difference from the much more massive and synchronous clonic movements can be used to diagnostic advantage. Although most eye-witnesses may not be able to describe the movements they have seen in much detail, they are often able to choose between the two types of movement, if a doctor mimics them. It should be noted that jerking movements probably do not occur in 90% of all syncope attacks: in fainting blood donors, the movements were only seen in about 12% of patients. The extreme and very sudden cessation of blood flow in the mess trick may account for the difference.

There are additional aspects that may help to ascribe jerks to either syncope or epilepsy. In syncope, jerks follow the fall, and never precede it, as may occur in epilepsy. If the jerks are unilateral at any moment during the attack, epilepsy is more likely than syncope. And finally, if the jerks start before consciousness is lost, epilepsy is quite likely (Tables 17.2–17.6 list a series of diagnostic clues).

Triggers in syncope and epilepsy

Epileptic attacks are not provoked by evident triggers. However, certain types of epilepsy, such as absences and complex partial seizures, tend not to appear during times of high activity. In contrast, many types of syncope are related to specific circumstances or triggers. For instance, the triggers that evoke the abnormal reflex in classic "vasovagal" syncope are well known. These may include pain, fear or anxiety. Only syncope due to arrhythmia regularly occurs under various circumstances without any recognizable common ground; in fact, this lack should alert the physician to think of arrhythmia (provided syncope is likelier than epilepsy on other grounds).

Table 17.2 History in transient loss of consciousness: events prior to the attack. These items have been gathered from several sources, and were ordered according to the course of events in an attack, ending with antecedent disorders. Note that for most of the items not enough information is available to evaluate their utility in terms of sensitivity and specificity.

Posture	
Lying	Reflex syncope and autonomic failure less likely, otherwise all possible causes
Standing	Reflex syncope and autonomic failure (in that case occurrence related to duration of standing)
Activity	
Standing up	Autonomic failure (in that case occurrence related to duration of standing)
Micturition, defecation	Reflex syncope
Protracted coughing	Reflex syncope
Swallowing	Reflex syncope including carotid sinus hypersensitivity
Predisposing factors	
After a meal	Autonomic failure, particularly in the elderly
Head movements, pressure on the neck, shaving	Carotid sinus hypersensitivity
Fear, pain, stress	Reflex syncope (classic vasovagal variant)
During physical exercise	Cardiac: structural cardiopulmonary disease
Directly after cessation of physical exercise	Autonomic failure
During exercise of the arms	Steal syndrome
Palpitations	Cardiac: arrhythmia
Startling (e.g., alarm clock)	Prolonged QT syndrome
Seeing flashing light	Epilepsy with photosensitivity
Sleep deprivation	Epilepsy
None; attacks appear to occur randomly	Epilepsy or cardiac: arrhythmia
Laughter	Cataplexy
Heat	Reflex syncope, autonomic failure

Table 17.3 History in transient loss of consciousness: events at the onset of the attack.

Nausea, sweating, pallor	"Autonomic activation": reflex syncope
Pain in shoulders, neck ("coat-hanger pattern")	Ischemia of local muscles: autonomic failure
Rising sensation from abdomen, unpleasant smell or taste, or other phenomena specific to subject but recurring over attacks	Epileptic aura

Table 17.4 History in transient loss of consciousness: events during the attack.

Fall

Keeling over, stiff	Tonic phase epilepsy, rarely syncope
Flaccid collapse	Syncope (all variants)

Movements*

Beginning before the fall	Epilepsy
Beginning after the fall	Epilepsy, syncope
Symmetric, synchronous	Epilepsy
Asymmetric, asynchronous	Syncope, may be epilepsy
Beginning at onset of unconsciousness	Epilepsy
Beginning after onset of unconsciousness	Syncope
Lasting less than about 15 sec	Syncope more likely than epilepsy
Lasting for 30 sec to minutes	Epilepsy
Restricted to one limb or one side	Epilepsy

Other aspects

Automatisms (chewing, smacking, blinking)	Epilepsy
Cyanotic face	Epilepsy
Eyes open	Epilepsy as likely as syncope
Tongue bitten	Epilepsy
Head consistently turned to one side	Epilepsy
Incontinence	Epilepsy as likely as syncope

* The word "clonic" is in everyday use restricted to epilepsy, while the word "myoclonus" is used for the movements in syncope as well as for certain types of epilepsy and to describe postanoxic movements (perhaps these share the same pathophysiology with syncopal myoclonus). The word "convulsions" is best reserved for epilepsy. "Myoclonic jerks" has little connotation with a specific cause, and is preferable to avoid jumping to conclusions.

Table 17.5 History in transient loss of consciousness: events after the attack.

Nausea, sweating, pallor	"Autonomic activation": syncope
Clearheaded immediately on regaining consciousness	Syncope, may occur in epilepsy
Confused during minutes after regaining consciousness	Epilepsy
Aching muscles (not to be confused with local bruises)	Epilepsy
Palpitations	Cardiac: arrhythmia
Chest pain	Cardiac: ischemia

"Reflex epilepsy" is often triggered by specific stimuli. The most common type is visually induced epilepsy: repeated visual stimuli may provoke an attack. A classical example is the sun flickering through the trees, but video games may be more relevant now. Non-specific startling sounds may also cause epilepsy. Finally, there is a wide array of other triggers that may induce epilepsy; this includes music (often restricted to a specific song), mental activity (again often restricted to a highly specific activity, such as arithmetic), hot water baths, eating, reading, etc. Usually, it takes repeated occurrences of such events for patients and doctors to become aware of the association. Most

Table 17.6 History in transient loss of consciousness: antecedent disorders.

Recent start or change of medication	Autonomic failure, may be arrhythmia
History of heart disease	Cardiac: arrhythmia or structural cardiac disease
Parkinsonism	Autonomic failure (primary type)
History of epilepsy	Epilepsy
Psychiatric history	May be psychogenic, but remember to check for autonomic failure due to medication!
Occurrence of sudden death in family members	Arrhythmia, specifically prolonged QT syndrome
Metabolic disorders (e.g., diabetes)	Real, non-circulatory transient loss of consciousness or autonomic failure (secondary)
Use of medication (antihypertensives, antiangina, antidepressives, phenothiazines, antiarrhythmics, diuretics)	Autonomic failure due to medication or hypovolemia; arrhythmia

triggers that can evoke reflex epilepsy do not evoke any type of syncope, and should therefore not cause much diagnostic confusion. One exception may be important: startling auditory stimuli may both cause epilepsy and arrhythmia in the prolonged QT syndrome; both conditions are very rare, though.

Steal syndrome

"Steal" refers to the condition in which a stenosis or occlusion of an artery causes such a low blood pressure beyond the stenosis that blood flow is diverted from another artery to flow into the low-pressure region. This presupposes that there are pre-existing connections between the "donor" artery and the poststenotic "acceptor" artery. The best-known example is a stenosis of the subclavian artery, in which the poststenotic artery receives an additional blood supply through the ipsilateral vertebral artery. Blood in that artery then flows down instead of upwards. Blood flows into that vertebral artery through the basilar artery, itself supplied through either the other vertebral artery or, through Willis' circle, through the carotid system.

Do "steal syndromes" cause syncope? This is certainly possible, as the vertebrobasilar system may be hard pressed to keep both the arm and the brainstem and occipital lobes supplied with blood. Indeed, symptoms attributed to vertebrobasilar steal include "vertigo", diplopia, blurred vision and cranial nerve dysfunction, as well as "syncope or drop attacks". Strictly speaking, TLOC resulting from steal should not be labeled as "syncope", as it is not due to a *global* but to a *regional* cerebral hypoperfusion. If there are several such signs or symptoms, it is not difficult to implicate the brainstem as the culprit, paving the way for the diagnosis. It is however, less clear how often an isolated TLOC without any brainstem signs or symptoms results from a steal phenomenon. The following considerations may help.

A blood pressure difference between the arms or complaints of claudication of one arm may point towards the presence of a steal phenomenon. However the presence of "steal" does not mean that any transient ischemic attacks (TIAs) or TLOC may be ascribed to it. In fact, slightly more than half (54%) of patients with a proven steal phenomenon have no clinical symptoms at all. And of the patients who do, only about one half have symptoms restricted to the vertebrobasilar region; the rest have carotid or combined symptoms. Pathologic and longitudinal studies have shown that infarctions of the vertebrobasilar artery apparently do not or hardly ever occur in this condition, meaning that it may be seen as a rather benign condition. It has gradually become clear that TIAs in a patient with steal only occur if there is atherosclerosis in other extracranial arteries as well. Physicians should therefore be wary of ascribing any TIA to a documented steal phenomenon. This holds true especially if the TIA involves the carotid territory.

In short, the chances that TLOC without any brainstem signs are due to subclavian steal are probably very small. Having said that, complaints may be ascribed to steal with more likelihood if they are clearly associated with exercise of one arm; under such circumstances the increased demands of the arm may decrease brainstem flow to below critical levels. Note that this concerns the left arm much more often than the right.

Apparent transient loss of consciousness

Whether this category can mimic syncope largely depends on the quality of the account of the events, as given by the patient or an eye-witness. Two factors are particularly important for history-taking: true loss of consciousness is absolutely incompatible with actively staying upright, and must be associated with amnesia for the event. Here, we will discuss disorders in which loss of consciousness is not present although it may appear to be so, as well as some conditions commonly but incorrectly thought to be accompanied by loss of consciousness. We will discuss cataplexy, psychiatric causes, TIAs and drop attacks.

Cataplexy

The symptom cataplexy occurs for all practical purposes only in the context of the disease narcolepsy. Although cataplexy is not widely known or recognized, it is not particularly rare. Cataplexy refers to loss of muscle tone due to emotions, particularly laughter. In contrast to vasovagal syncope pain, fear and anxiety are not strong triggers. Startle may provoke cataplexy, but over a series of attacks it is never the only trigger, or the most common one. According to most textbooks, patients suddenly slump to the ground with complete paralysis. Partial attacks are, however, more common. These can be restricted to dropping of the jaw and sagging or nodding of the head. Attacks may develop slowly enough to allow the patient to stagger and break the fall before he or she comes to lie on the floor. Complete attacks look like syncope in that the unfortunate patient is unable to respond at all, although he or she is completely conscious and aware of what is going on. The presence of consciousness can in fact only be assessed later through the absence of amnesia. Although narcolepsy may start with cataplexy, this is rare. Faced with laughter-related attacks, physicians should ask for the presence of excessive daytime sleepiness, narcolepsy's main symptom. When in doubt, refer to a neurologist: the condition is well treatable.

Psychiatry and syncope (see also Chapter 13)

Although the term "psychogenic syncope" may be found in the literature, authors probably mean "psychogenic pseudo-syncope". Otherwise there would have to be a way to shut down cerebral perfusion through a mental process (none exists). In a broader sense, "psychogenic" should be treated with much caution when dealing with epidemiologic or individual studies on real or apparent TLOC. Often, the diagnosis of "psychogenic" relies on exclusion of other causes rather than on a positive ground or on a careful psychiatric examination. Estimates of how often attacks are "psychogenic" should therefore be viewed with caution. On this somewhat shaky basis, we may discuss three entities touching on psychiatry.

Pseudo-unconsciousness

This is not a common term. Here, it denotes that patients act as if they are unconsciousness while they are not. This is not uncommon in emergency rooms. In the *DSM-IV*, the standard psychiatric diagnostic manual, a distinction is made between three entities. In "conversion disorder" patients show unexplained somatic symptoms at a time when psychologic factors are also apparent. In the past, it was thought this action was due to represented suppressed problems, was not under voluntary control, and that patients were unaware of the psychogenic origin of the complaint; the *DSM-IV* now shies away from any explanation (see also Chapter 13). A "factitious disorder" means that patients intentionally pretend to be ill in order to assume the sick role; in "malingering" they do the same, but to gain some other advantage, such as avoiding some task or duty. These three forms look alike from a somatic point of view, so we will focus on how to distinguish them from true unconsciousness.

Usually, a state of pseudo-unconsciousness will probably have lasted too long for it to be confused with syncope, so the differential diagnosis is one of coma rather than of syncope. Still, similar states may occur during consultation or tilt-table testing, so it is important to know a few tell-tale features that help differentiate them from true unconsciousness. First of all, there should be no gross abnormalities during a neurologic examination, except for a lack of responsiveness. Although such patients lie relaxed with their eyes shut, their muscle tone differs from that of truly unconscious subjects, resulting in a non-flaccid posture of the limbs, recognizable to trained eyes. There may be a tendency to sudden and active closure of the eyes when these are opened passively. When a lifted limb is let go it may hesitate shortly in midair before it starts to fall. Likewise, the patient's hand, held above the face and let go, will not drop onto the face but will just miss it. There may be reflexive gaze movements, or the eyes may be turned upwards, downwards or consistently away from the observer. Such patients may show an incredible ability to suppress any response to pain, so this has little value for the diagnosis. A slightly more invasive test concerns ice-water irrigation of the ears, producing an eye deviation in comatose subjects but a lively nystagmus in awake ones. Note that "tricks" as described here should not be used to hold a patient in contempt as a fraud, but simply to restore communication, allowing the problem to be addressed. Remarks made to others in the patient's hearing range that such states "usually pass quickly" may be more helpful than a confrontational approach.

During a tilt-table test apparent unconsciousness with intact blood pressure and heart rate may indicate a feigned or conversive response. However, there are other ways to lose consciousness than through abnormalities of the systemic circulation, so this is not enough to establish pseudo-unconsciousness. This requires features as outlined above or, even better, the documentation that there are no functional cerebral disturbances on an electroencephalogram (EEG): if the EEG does not change while consciousness is apparently being lost, true unconsciousness is ruled out.

"Hyperventilation"

"Hyperventilation" does not equal the "hyperventilation syndrome", and secondly, the "hyperventilation syndrome" does not occur at all in the *DSM-IV*. "Hyperventilation" simply refers to breathing more than metabolic needs warrant. This leads to a series of physiologic events, including hypocapnia, constriction of cerebral vessels and reduced cerebral blood flow. As such, the act of hyperventilation could certainly contribute to syncope, or theoretically even cause it. Lightheadedness and tingling fingers or toes may with good reason be seen as physiologic manifestations of breathing too much, and do not necessarily indicate psychologic factors. This does not hold for a large variety of other complaints, such as anxiety, fear or various other somatic-sounding phenomena, that may occur together under stressful circumstances and that are often bundled together as the "hyperventilation syndrome".

Within the term "hyperventilation syndrome" is the assumption that hyperventilation is evoked by stress, and that the resulting overbreathing and hypocapnia cause the complaints. However, a series of intriguing studies have called this concept into question. Experiments in which hyperventilating subjects were supplied with extra CO_2 to make them normocapnic suggest that many complaints were in fact not linked to hypocapnia. The matter has not been resolved completely, however. Overbreathing can at least contribute to the complaints, even if it is not at their root. The particular set of complaints may be found in the *DSM-IV* under "panic disorder".

Can hyperventilation cause syncope? As noted above, the resulting reduction of cerebral perfusion might contribute to syncope, but it is at present unknown whether or not hyperventilation on its own can cause syncope. An argument against this is that one of the first effects of impaired consciousness would probably be that voluntary control over ventilation is lost. Autonomic circuits, taking over, would immediately end hyperventilation and thereby restore consciousness. Theoretically, syncope could still ensue if this resumption of normal control would lag significantly behind the constriction of cerebral vessels. A perhaps likelier association between hyperventilation and syncope is that the anxiety in a panic attack evokes both hyperventilation as a stress response, as well as a vasovagal reflex syncope.

Lacking any clear evidence that hyperventilation causes syncope on its own, it seems prudent to consider hyperventilation as a physiologic phenomenon that may increase the chances of syncope due to other processes. Secondly, keep in mind that the term "hyperventilation syndrome" may be a misnomer because that particular constellation of complaints does not necessarily require the act of hyperventilation.

Syncope in psychiatric patients

Non-psychiatrists may tend to label complaints of patients with a psychiatric history as "psychogenic". As we have seen, the three psychiatric disorders resembling syncope are conversion, factitious disorders and malingering. There is no reason to suppose that these occur overly often in major psychiatric diseases such as depression, schizophrenia and bipolar disorder, any more than they would in many somatic diseases. Note that true syncope may, however, occur with increased frequency in these disorders, due to medication causing orthostatic hypotension, i.e., autonomic failure. Main culprits are phenothiazines, tricyclic antidepressives, and monoamine oxidase inhibitors. Rather than turning to the "blind-alley" approach of labeling attacks in such patients as "psychogenic", a careful history should determine whether the attacks fit the pattern of syncope in autonomic failure. If so, a revision of medication may be called for.

Transient ischemic attacks

As a rule, TIAs do not cause attacks of transient loss of consciousness. The majority of TIAs affect the territory of one carotid artery. When this happens, a large variety of neurologic functions may be lost, but consciousness is not foremost among them. As has been said, loss of consciousness points to a severe loss of function of the brainstem or a very large portion of the cortex. In patients with a massive stroke of one hemisphere and additional damage, consciousness may indeed be lowered, so we may theoretically expect that this can also occur in a TIA. This is not a common presentation however, and the accompanying impressive loss of hemispheric function with hemiparesis as the most obvious feature rules out any chance that this can be mistaken for syncope, in which only consciousness is lost, and no other neurologic function.

The same reasoning applies for vertebrobasilar TIAs. Here, consciousness may be supposed to be affected more often than in a carotid TIA, but it is not likely that loss of consciousness would be the only feature of such TIAs. Ataxia, dysarthria, paresis, hemianopia and a variety of other signs predominate in vertebrobasilar TIAs. This knowledge should affect the choice of any additional investigations in patients with TLOC without accompanying neurologic deficits: ultrasound studies of cerebral vessels are not indicated.

Drop attacks

The term "drop attack" is one of the vaguest and least helpful in medical terminology. A conservative approach to deal with it would be to reserve it for a specific clinical phenomenon without attributing any specific cause to it. The phenomenon would then be a very short-lasting attack in which a patient suddenly falls without any warning, and without any other feature whatsoever. The attacks last for too short a time for patients to be certain whether there was any loss of consciousness. Commonly, they remember landing on the floor, so any loss of conscience would have to be extremely short, if it existed at all. Apart from possible injuries and being startled, patients have nothing else to tell about the attacks. When used in this sense, a variety of disorders come into play as possible causes of this phenomenon. Unfortunately, many researchers use the term as a substitute for a particular cause. Several will be discussed.

First, the term "drop attacks" was coined in 1974 to describe a syndrome in which the individual "dropped" without loss of consciousness. The attacks occurred in middle-aged people, and more often in women. Patients often bruised their knees. There were no other features, and patients did not develop other signs or symptoms. This may be the best use of the term. Second, the term is also used to describe "astatic" or "atonic" epileptic seizures. In such cases, the attacks may last longer than described above. They are accompanied by specific EEG abnormalities. These attacks occur in the context of myoclonic attacks in young children. Third, "drop attacks" was used to describe episodes of falling in patients with Ménière's disease. Short-lived disturbances of the vestibular system may have caused sudden dysequilibrium, described as being "pushed" by patients. Finally, some authors appear to use "drop attacks" simply as a substitute for unexplained falling. In this sense the term has no advantage over "falling" itself, which at least carries no connotation of any specific cause.

Disentangling the clues: considerations for various specialists

For medical specialists, it is daunting, if not impossible, to step over the borders of one's specialty and to consider a differential diagnosis mixing neurologic, cardiac, psychiatric and internal medicine disorders. In truth, however, this conundrum does not occur that often, suggesting that the initial assignment to a specialty-based category usually works well. When errors are made, the patient will usually have moved on to a specialist, who now has to move up one step in the hierarchy of disorders, i.e., from epilepsy or syncope to TLOC.

   The best approach is to see whether anything was missed in the history of the TLOC episodes. A thorough step-by-step history of as many attacks as possible needs to be taken from both patients and any eye-witnesses. To help with this, pointers from various sources have been compiled (Tables 17.2–17.6). More specific advice may be directed at neurologists and cardiologists, who often see each others' patients. Note that both have a similar problem: in episodic cardiac rhythm disturbances as well as in epilepsy interictal abnormalities need not be present on the ECG or the EEG. The problem is not unlike fishing: you can only be certain that there are fish when one is caught; until then, the presence of fish cannot be excluded. To avoid misunderstanding test results, the presence or absence of any clinical attacks during long-term ECG or EEG recordings should always be mentioned in the reports.

What if you are a neurologist?

The most obvious mistake in this case is that a patient with syncope was referred as having epilepsy. The initial judgement was probably to blame for the mistake, in which myoclonic jerks were interpreted as epileptic clonic movements. Note that the difference can indeed be difficult to distinguish, and that an eye-witness may understandably be hard pressed to give a detailed description of a very impressive and apparently life-threatening event. When a neurologist suspects syncope, a division into the main categories must be made. Reflex syncope and autonomic failure in the form of orthostatic hypotension do not necessarily require cardiologic expertise, but the one form that must not be missed is syncope due to underlying cardiac disease, in view of the high associated mortality. Neurologists should therefore know how to differentiate between the main categories (Table 17.2). The difficulty increases if there was only one event and if there are no clear epileptiform EEG abnormalities. As an erroneous diagnosis of epilepsy may have profound effects on quality of life, withholding antiepileptic medication is warranted, at least until more evidence in favor of epilepsy is gained. If there are mild epileptiform abnormalities, one should keep in mind that there is a chance of about 1% that the EEG is falsely abnormal, and that there are several normal EEG phenomena that may be mistaken as "epileptiform". In case of repeated attacks history-taking should focus on a trigger pattern, and on features such as postictal confusion, that may help differentiate between types of TLOC. The absence of any recognizable trigger pattern is compatible with epilepsy, but should also raise suspicions of rhythm disturbances.

What if you are a cardiologist?

Here, the reverse situation applies: as it is gradually becoming better known that syncope may be associated with myoclonic jerks, there is now a chance that epilepsy may be mistaken for syncope. Table 17.2 may be helpful in selecting a proper cause. In the case of a single attack, the history should determine what to do. If there are features suggesting epilepsy, such as prolonged confusion, referral is warranted. In the case of repeated attacks a pattern should be sought. If none is found epilepsy is possible, and should be investigated.

What if you are an emergency room physician?

As doctors in emergency rooms are among the first to see a patient with TLOC, they are less likely than others further up the chain to suffer from others' faulty diagnoses. A possible danger is relying too much on overly quick associations made by passers-by or paramedical personnel. The real challenge for the emergency room physician is not to reach a faulty diagnosis oneself, and in this respect the greatest danger is to jump too quickly to a specific syndrome instead of starting at the root, i.e., TLOC. It is probably wise to consider diagnostic actions from three angles: always expect the common (reflex syncope, epilepsy); be wary of the dangerous (cardiac syncope); and consider whether any tests need to be carried out now or after referral.

What if you are a general practitioner?

General practitioners face the same problem as emergency room physicians, with two differences: they do not have a hospital's array of tests at their immediate disposal, and see more patients in whom no further action is necessary. The task of correctly picking out the dangerous conditions is therefore less easy, while the danger of letting them go undetected is greater. More than any other physician, general practitioners must therefore be skilled in taking a detailed TLOC history.

What if you are a pediatrician?

The array of disorders causing TLOC in children differs from that in adults. Cardiac causes are rare, and the types of epilepsy affecting children differ from those in adults. Some forms of epilepsy, such as absence epilepsy or Rolandic attacks, hardly ever affect adults. The terminology of syncope is even more confusing in children than in adults. There are two types of breath-holding spells, "pallid" and "cyanotic". "Pallid breath-holding spells", also called "reflex anoxic seizures", are the same form of reflex syncope that is called vasovagal syncope in adolescents and adults. The nature of cyanotic breath-holding spells is not quite clear; hyperventilation or a Valsalva maneuver may be to blame.

In small children, common triggers for reflex syncope are a fall or bumping the head. The resulting unconsciousness does not ensue immediately, proving that it was not due to brain trauma but to emotion caused by the attack. As in adults, the presence of a trigger is very important in deciding between epilepsy and syncope.

Summary

"Syncope" does not equal "transient loss of consciousness". In undetermined attacks, "unexplained syncope" limits thinking to syncope, while "TLOC" does not. Further, all that shakes is not epilepsy. While syncope is commonly triggered, epilepsy is commonly not. Beware of medication-induced orthostatic hypotension in subjects with a psychiatric history.

"Psychogenic syncope" is an impossibility, but "psychogenic pseudo-syncope" certainly occurs. The complaints in the "hyperventilation syndrome" do not necessarily require the act of hyperventilation. If loss of consciousness is not accompanied by signs or symptoms suggesting dysfunction of the brainstem or a hemisphere, then a TIA or steal syndrome is highly unlikely.

Further reading

Commission on classification and terminology of the international league against epilepsy. Proposal for revised classification of epilepsies and epileptic syndromes. *Epilepsia* 1989; 30: 389–399.

DSM-IV. Diagnostic and statistical manual of mental disorders. American Psychiatric Association. Washington 1994.

Hornsveld HK, Garssen B, Dop MJ, van Spiegel PI, de Haes JC. Double-blind placebo-controlled study of the hyperventilation provocation test and the validity of the hyperventilation syndrome. *Lancet* 1996; 348: 154–1588.

Lempert T, Bauer M, Schmidt D. Syncope: a videometric analysis of 56 episodes of transient cerebral hypoxia. *Ann Neurol* 1994; 36: 233–237.

Taylor CL, Selman WR, Ratcheson RA. Steal affecting the central nervous system. *Neurosurg* 2002; 50: 679–689.

CHAPTER 18

Whom to treat

Michele Brignole, Rose Anne Kenny

Introduction

Treatment objectives for the "syncope patient" may be classified into prevention of syncopal recurrences, and diminution of mortality risk. Multiple factors affect the need for recommending the specific treatment strategy selected for each individual. In this regard, treatment may be broadly viewed as education, non-pharmacologic and pharmacologic treatments directed at syncope susceptibility (including addressing underlying disease state), and lifestyle recommendations.

Goals

The goals of this chapter are to highlight:
- factors determining need for treatment for prevention of syncope recurrences;
- the objective of therapy in various syncope diagnostic categories; and
- issues affecting the "aggressiveness" of treatment, including the need for addressing underlying disease issues.

Factors affecting decision regarding need for treatment

The need for initiating prophylactic treatment varies depending on specific clinical circumstances. The most important of these are:
- level of certainty that the etiology of the symptoms is known;
- an estimate of the likelihood that syncope will recur;
- the individual's anticipated syncope-associated mortality risk which is, for the most part, determined by the nature and severity of underlying cardiac and cardiovascular disease;
- the occurrence of, or potential risk for, physical or emotional injury associated with recurrent faints;
- the implications of syncope recurrence on occupation and avocation (i.e., individual economic and lifestyle issues);
- the public health risk, such as in the case of motor vehicle operators, pilots, etc.; and
- an assessment of the effectiveness, safety and potential adverse effects associated with proposed therapies (in particular given comorbidities in the patient being evaluated).

Specific conditions

Neurally mediated reflex syncopal syndromes

Since neurally mediated syncope carries virtually no direct mortality risk, the treatment goals: are directed almost exclusively toward primarily prevention of both symptom recurrence and associated injuries and improved quality of life.

There are no concrete guidelines regarding who merits treatment beyond education and reassurance in this group of patients. Treatment is probably not necessary for patients who have sustained a single syncope, are not having syncope in a high-risk setting, and who are not at excessive risk of sustaining significant injury (e.g., fractures). Conversely, patients with multiple faints over an extended period of time (> 6 months) are likely to have future recurrences, and treatment may then be warranted. Patients who present with significant injury (e.g., subdural hemorrhage) associated with a single or rare faint need special consideration. While it may be true that the injury was simply "bad luck" (i.e., just happened to occur in an injury-prone location), the seriousness of the event create extreme concern for the patient and/or family members.

Patients who have syncope in a "high-risk" setting (e.g., commercial vehicle driver, machine operator, pilot, competitive athlete) merit specific consideration for treatment. These individuals need earlier and more aggressive treatment to reduce risk of injury to themselves or others. Commercial pilots pose a particularly difficult problem in this regard as regulatory agencies vary in interpretation of treatment success. Consequently, it has been very difficult for these individuals to return to active employment. A consensus needs to be developed with regard to treatment end-points in such settings, but this is a long way from being achieved.

Orthostatic syncope

The treatment goals in these individuals are directed to prevention of symptom recurrence and associated injuries, and to improve quality of life. Many of these patients are in older age groups and/or are more frail due to the presence of multiple concomitant medical conditions. Iatrogenic factors, as well as poor diet and fluid intake may play a key role in triggering symptoms in such cases.

Syncope due to symptomatic orthostatic hypotension should be treated in all patients. In many instances treatment entails only modification of drug treatment for concomitant conditions. Thus, if new-onset orthostatic syncope can be reasonably attributed to a drug being taken by the individual then its withdrawal should suffice. However, clinical follow-up is still warranted.

Cardiac arrhythmias as primary cause

Treatment goals are prevention of symptom recurrence, improved quality of life and reduction of mortality risk.

Syncope due to cardiac arrhythmias must receive treatment appropriate to the cause in all patients in whom it is life-threatening and when there is a high risk of injury. The latter is often the case in elderly or frail individuals, those in whom warning is minimal or absent, and those whose employment might result in physical injury to themselves or others.

Structural cardiac or cardiopulmonary disease

Treatment goals are prevention of symptom recurrence, and reduction of mortality risk. There is consensus that the following should be treated:

- Syncope accompanied by severe physical injury, involving a motor vehicle or other accident, or occurring in a "high-risk" setting (e.g., commercial vehicle driver, machine operator, pilot, commercial painter, competitive athlete), or which may result in substantial economic hardship such as due to loss of employment or employment opportunity, or restricted lifestyle.
- Syncope associated with critical valvular or coronary artery stenosis, hypertrophic obstructive cardiomyopathy (HOCM), arrhythmogenic ventricular dysplasia (ARVD) and/or life-threatening ventricular tachyarrhythmias.

There is less certainty whether to treat patients with recurrent "near-syncopal" spells or "dizziness", with an ejection fraction (EF) < 35%, but in whom the cause of syncope is unproven. Treatment is not indicated in cases of single (or infrequent) syn-copal episode(s), without injury and not in a high-risk setting, in which there is evidence of tachyarrhythmia but there are no economic or lifestyle concerns, or where the patient is considered "end-stage" due to other life-threatening medical issues.

Cerebrovascular

The goals of treatment of syncope associated with cerebrovascular disease (see Chapter 14, Part 5) are aimed at preventing stroke and improving quality of life.

Subclavian steal is the only commonly recognized condition in this group. There are no well defined treatment indications, but intervention seems appropriate when the condition is severe enough to cause clinically important symptoms such as syncope or near-syncope.

Recurrent syncope is uncommon in patients even with bilateral critical carotid artery stenosis, or with vertebrobasilar disease. Treatment of these conditions may be indicated to prevent stroke, but a "syncope" indication would be extremely rare.

Miscellaneous syncope-like conditions

Disorders in this category are not true syncope (see Chapter 17), but are part of the differential diagnosis. Treatment goals are primarily aimed at improved quality of life.

Psychiatric disturbances

The importance of psychiatric disturbances as syncope mimics lies in the fact that they are both very common and difficult to diagnose. Often, the diagnosis only materializes after considerable time and unproductive laboratory testing. If recurrent "syncope-like" symptoms are a feature of the patient's presentation then psychiatric referral for treatment is indicated.

Seizure disorders

Seizure disorders are part of the differential diagnosis of transient loss of consciousness, but are rare as causes of syncope. Frontal lobe partial complex seizures may be misdiagnosed as true syncope by virtue of their tendency to be abrupt in onset, brief, and often unassociated with postictal confusion. Temporal lobe seizures may also mimic (or possibly trigger) vasovagal syncope. Conventional seizure therapy under the care of a neurologist is appropriate.

Metabolic disturbances

Apart from hyperventilation resulting in loss of consciousness, metabolic disturbances (e.g., hypoglycemic coma, hypoxemia) causing loss of consciousness are best considered as syncope mimics by virtue of the fact that they are not typically self-limited. Treatment is indicated in all cases, and may require referral to a specialist in internal medicine.

Intoxication

Various agents, most commonly alcohol, may induce alterations of consciousness that mimic syncope. As a rule, however, the episode is relatively long-lasting, and not immediately reversible as is usually expected in true syncope.

Summary

Treatment of syncope patients is critically dependent on establishing the correct diagnosis, and understanding the patient's overall health condition and social circumstances. Apart from education regarding syncope which should be universally provided, various specific issues determine the need for further treatment steps. Certain of these considerations have been summarized in this chapter. More detailed analysis is found in the previous chapters dealing with individual conditions in detail.

Further reading

Brignole M, Alboni P, Benditt DG *et al.* Guidelines on management (diagnosis and treatment) of syncope. *Eur Heart J* 2001; 22: 1256–1306.

Kapoor W. Evaluation and outcome of patients with syncope. *Medicine* 1990; 69: 160–175.

Sheldon R, Rose S, Ritchie D *et al.* Historical criteria that distinguish syncope from seizures. *J Am Coll Cardiol* 2002; 40: 142–148.

Selected references published since 1990

(With the exception of the sections entitled "Guidelines/task force statements/ consensus statements" and "Classic articles", the editors have restricted the references to those published since the beginning of 1990. The reader will find a comprehensive bibliography in the ESC Syncope Task Force Guidelines Statement (*Eur Heart J* 2001), and additional articles are noted at the end of each chapter labelled "Further reading".)

Guidelines/task force statements/consensus statements

Commission on classification and terminology of the international league against epilepsy. Proposal for revised classification of epilepsies and epileptic syndromes. *Epilepsia* 1989; 30: 389–399.

Breithardt G, Cain ME, El-Sherif N *et al.* Standards for analysis of ventricular late potentials using high resolution or signal-averaged electrocardiography. A statement by a Task Force Committee between the European Society of Cardiology, the American Heart Association and the American College of Cardiology. *Eur Heart J* 1991; 12: 473–480.

DSM IV. Diagnostic and statistical manual of mental disorders. American Psychiatric Association. Washington 1994.

The Consensus Committee of the American Autonomic Society and the American Academy of Neurology. Consensus statement on the definition of orthostatic hypotension, pure autonomic failure, and multiple system atrophy. *Neurology* 1996; 46: 1470.

Benditt DG, Ferguson DW, Grubb BP *et al.* Tilt table testing for assessing syncope. ACC expert consensus document. *J Am Coll Cardiol* 1996; 28: 263–275.

Epstein AE, Miles WM, Benditt DG *et al.* Personal and public safety issues related to arrhythmias that may affect consciousness: implications for regulation and physician recommendations. *Circulation* 1996; 94: 1147–1166.

Royal College of Physicians. Adults with poorly controlled epilepsy: Clinical guidelines for treatment and practical tools for aiding epilepsy management. July 1997. ISBN 1 86016 062 X. Code 15113 002.

Linzer M, Yang E, Estes M *et al.* Clinical Guideline. Diagnosing syncope. Part 1: Value of history, clinical examination, and electrocardiography. *Ann Intern Med* 1997; 126: 989–996.

Linzer M, Yang E, Estes M *et al.* Clinical Guideline. Diagnosing syncope. Part 2: Unexplained syncope. *Ann Intern Med* 1997; 127: 76–86.

Petch MC. Driving and heart disease. Task Force Report. Prepared on behalf of the ESC Task Force. *Eur Heart J* 1998; 19: 1165–1177.

Gilman S, Low PA, Quinn N *et al.* Consensus statement on the diagnosis of multiple system atrophy. *J Neurol Sci* 1999; 163; 94–98.

Crawford MH, Bernstein SJ, Deedwania PC *et al.* ACC/AHA Guidelines for Ambulatory Electrocardiography. *J Am Coll Cardiol* 1999; 34: 912–948. (Executive summary and recommendations. *Circulation* 1999; 100: 886–893.)

Haverkamp W, Breithardt G, Camm AJ *et al.* The potential for QT prolongation and proarrhythmia by non-antiarrhythmic drugs: clinical and regulatory implications. Report on a Policy Conference of the European Society of Cardiology. *Eur Heart J* 2000; 21: 1216–1231.

Brignole M, Alboni P, Benditt DG *et al.* Guidelines on management (diagnosis and treatment) of syncope. *Eur Heart J* 2001; 22: 1256–1306.

Guideline for the prevention of falls in older persons. American Geriatrics Society, British Geriatrics Society, and American Academy of Orthopaedic Surgeons Panel on Falls Prevention. *J Am Geriatr Soc* 2001; 49(5): 664–672.

Gregoratos G, Abrams J, Epstein AE *et al.* ACC/AHA/NASPE 2002 guideline update for implantation of cardiac pacemakers and antiarrhythmia devices: summary article. *Circulation* 2002; 106: 2145–2161.

Flink R, Pedersen B, Guekht AB *et al.* Guidelines for the use of EEG methodology in the diagnosis of epilepsy. International League Against Epilepsy: commission report. Commission on European Affairs: Subcommission on European Guidelines. *Acta Neurol Scand* 2002; 106: 1–7.

Priori SG, Aliot E, Blomstrom-Ludqvist C *et al.* Task Force on Sudden Cardiac Death. European Society of Cardiology. Summary of recommmendations. *Europace* 2002; 4: 3–18.

Bernstein AD, Daubert JC, Fletcher *et al.* The revised NASPE/BPEG generic code for antibradycardia, adaptive-rate, and multisite pacing. *PACE* 2002; 25: 260–264.

Goldschlager N, Epstein AE, Grubb BP *et al.* Practice Guidelines subcommittee, NASPE. Etiologic considerations in the patient with syncope and an apparently normal heart. *Arch Int Med* 2003; 163: 151–162.

"Classic" articles

Maclean AR, Allen EV. Orthostatic hypotension and orthostatic tachycardia; treatment with the 'head-up' bed. *J Am Med Assoc* 1940; 115: 2162–2167.

Rossen R, Kabat H, Anderson JP. Acute arrest of cerebral circulation in man. *Arch Neurol Psychiatr* 1943; 50: 510–528.

Barcroft H, Edholm OG, McMichael J, Sharpey-Schafer EP. Posthaemorrhagic fainting. *Lancet* 1944; i: 489–491.

Sharpey-Schafer EP, Hayter CJ, Barlow ED. Mechanism of acute hypotension from fear and nausea. *Br Med J* 1958; 2: 878–880.

Johnson AM. Aortic stenosis, sudden death, and the left ventricular baroreceptors. *Br Heart J* 1971; 33: 1–5.

Goldreyer BN, Kastor JA, Kershbaum KL. The hemodynamic effects of induced supraventricular tachycardia in man. *Circulation* 1976; 54: 783–789.

Strangaard S. Autoregulation of cerebral blood flow in hypertensive patients: the modifying influence of prolonged antihypertensive treatment on the tolerance of acute drug induced hypotension. *Circulation* 1976; 53: 720–729.

Gann D, Tolentino A, Samet P. Electrophysiologic evaluation of elderly patients with sinus bradycardia. A long-term follow-up study. *Ann Intern Med* 1979; 90: 24–29.

Rushton JG, Stevens JC, Miller RH. Glossopharyngeal (vagoglossopharyngeal) neuralgia. A study of 217 cases. *Arch Neurol* 1981; 38: 21–205.

Ausubel K, Furman S. The pacemaker syndome. *Ann Intern Med* 1985; 103: 420.

Kapoor W, Karpf M, Maher Y *et al.* Syncope of unknown origin: the need for a more cost-effective approach to its diagnostic evaluation. *JAMA* 1982; 247: 2687–2691.

Savage DD, Corwin L, McGee DL *et al.* Epidemiologic features of isolated syncope: The Framingham Study. *Stroke* 1985; 16: 626–629.

Lipsitz LA, Pluchino FC, Wei JY, Rowe JW. Syncope in an elderly instituzionalized population: prevalence, incidence and associated risk. *Q J Med* 1985; 55: 45–54.

Huycke EC, Card HG, Sobol SM, Nguyen NX, Sung RJ. Postexertional cardiac asystole in a young man without organic heart disease. *Ann Intern Med* 1987; 106: 844–845.

Kenny RA, Ingram A, Bayliss J, Sutton R. Head-up tilt: a useful test for investigating unexplained syncope. *Lancet* 1986 Jun 14; 1: 1352–1355.

Rosenqvist M, Brandt J, Schuller H. Long-term pacing in sick sinus node disease: effects of stimulation mode on cardiovascular morbidity and mortality. *Am Heart J* 1988; 116: 16–22.

Bass EB, Elson JJ, Fogoros RN, Peterson J, Arena VC, Kapoor WN. Long-term prognosis of patients undergoing electrophysiologic studies for syncope of unknown origin. *Am J Cardiol* 1988; 62: 1186–1191.

Almquist A, Goldenberg IF, Milstein S *et al.* Provocation of bradycardia and hypotension by isoproterenol and upright posture in patients with unexplained syncope. *N Engl J Med* 1989 9; 320: 346–351.

Fujimura O, Yee R, Klein G, Sharma A, Boahene A. The diagnostic sensitivity of electrophysiologic testing in patients with syncope caused by transient bradycardia. *N Engl J Med* 1989; 321: 1703–1707.

Pathophysiology of syncope

Van Lieshout JJ, Wieling W, Karemaker JM, Eckberg D. The vasovagal response. *Clin Sci* 1991; 81: 575–586.

Leitch JW, Klein GJ, Yee R *et al.* Syncope associated with supraventricular tachycardia: An expression of tachycardia or vasomotor response. *Circulation* 1992; 85: 1064–1071.

Brignole M, Gianfranchi L, Menozzi C *et al.* Role of autonomic reflexes in syncope associated with paroxysmal atrial fibrillation. *J Am Coll Cardiol* 1993; 22: 1123–1129.

Alboni P, Menozzi C, Brignole M *et al.* An abnormal neural reflex plays a role in causing syncope. in sinus bradycardia. *J Am Coll Cardiol* 1993; 22: 1130–1134.

Rowell LB. *Human Cardiovascular Control*. New York, Oxford University Press, 1993.

Lempert T, Bauer M, Schmidt D. Syncope: A videometric analysis of 56 episodes of transient cerebral hypoxia. *Ann Neurol* 1994; 36: 233–237.

Hainsworth R, El Bedawi KM. Orthostatic tolerance in patients with unexplained syncope. *Clin Autonom Res* 1994; 4: 239–244.

Shannon RP, Wei JY, Rosa RM *et al.* The effect of age and sodium depletion on cardiovascular response to orthostasis. *Hypertension* 1986; 8: 438–443.

El-Sayed H, Hainsworth R. Relationship between plasma volume, carotid baroreceptor sensitivity and orthostatic tolerance. *Clin Sci* 1995; 88: 463–470.

Tea SH, Mansourati J, L'Heveder G, Mabin D, Blanc JJ. New insights into the pathophysiology of carotid sinus syndrome. *Circulation* 1996; 93: 1411–1416.

Blanc JJ, L'Heveder G, Mansourati J *et al.* Assessment of newly recognized association: carotid sinus hypersensitivity and denervation of sternocleidomastoid muscles. *Circulation* 1997; 95: 2548–2551.

Wieling W, van Lieshout JJ, ten Harkel ADJ. Dynamics of circulatory adjustments to head up tilt and tilt back in healthy and sympathetically denervated subjects. *Clin Sci* 1998; 94: 347–352.

Hainsworth R. Syncope and fainting: classification and pathophysiological basis. In: Mathias CJ, Bannister R eds. *Autonomic Failure. A Textbook of Clinical Disorders of the Autonomic Nervous System*, 4th edn. Oxford, Oxford University Press 1999 pp. 428–436.

Smit AAJ, Halliwill JR, Low PA, Wieling W. Topical Review. Pathophysiological basis of orthostatic hypotension in autonomic failure. *J Physiol* 1999; 519: 1–10.

Robertson RM, Medina E, Shah N, Furlan R, Mosqueda-Garcia R. Neurally mediated syncope: pathophysiology and implications for treatment. *Am J Med Sci* 1999; 317: 102–109.

Schondorf R, Wieling W. Vasoconstrictor reserve in neurally mediated syncope. *Clin Autonom Res* 2000; 10: 53–56.

Harms MPM, Collier W, Wieling W, Lenders JWM, Secher NH, van Lieshout JJ. Cerebral blood flow velocity and oxygenation in patients with neurogenic orthostatic hypotension during orthostic stress. *Stroke* 2000; 31: 1608–1614.

Omboni S, Smit AA, van Lieshout JJ *et al.* Mechanisms underlying the impairment in orthostatic intolerance after nocturnal recumbency in patients with autonomic failure. *Clin Sci* 2001; 101: 609–618.

Mathias CJ, Deguchi K, Schatz I. Observations on recurrent syncope and presyncope in 641 patients. *Lancet* 2001; 357: 348–353.

Mathias CJ. To stand on one's own legs. *Clin Med* 2002; 2: 237–245.

Mukai S, Lipsitz LA. Orthostatic hypotension. *Clin Geriatr Med* 2002; 18: 253–268.

Goldstein DS, Robertson D, Esler M, Straus SE, Eisenhofer G. Dysautonomias: Clinical disorders of the autonomic nervous system. *Ann Intern Med* 2002; 137: 753–763.

Wieling W, Halliwill JR, Karemaker JM. Orthostatic intolerance after space flight (editorial). *J Physiol* 2002; 538: 1.

Ermis C, Samniah N, Lurie KG *et al.* Adrenal/renal contribution to circulating norepinephrine in posturally induced neurally mediated reflex syncope. *Am J Cardiol* 2003; 91: 746–750.

Goldstein DS, Holmes C, Frank SM *et al.* Sympathoadrenal imbalance before neurocardiogenic syncope. *Am J Cardiol* 2003; 91: 53–58.

Epidemiology

Morichetti A, Astorino G. Epidemiological and clinical findings in 697 syncope events. *Min Med* 1998; 89: 211–220.

Lewis DA, Dhala A. Syncope in the pediatric patient. The cardiologist's perspective. *Pediatr Clin North Am* 1999; 46: 205–219.

Ammirati F, Colivicchi F, Santini M *et al.* Diagnosing syncope in clinical practice. Implementation of a simplified diagnostic algorithm in a multicentre prospective trial—the OESIL 2 study (Observatorio Epidemiologico della Sincope nel Lazio). *Eur Heart J* 2000; 21: 935–940.

Sarasin FP, Louis-Simonet M, Carballo D *et al.* Prospective evaluation of patients with syncope: a population-based study. *Am J Med* 2001; 111: 177–184.

Blanc J-J, L'Her C, Touiza A *et al.* Prospective evaluation and outcome of patients admitted for syncope over a 1 year period. *Eur Heart J* 2002; 23: 815–820.

Soteriades ES, Evans JC, Larson MG *et al.* Incidence and prognosis of syncope. *N Engl J Med* 2002; 347(12): 878–885.

Economics/social costs

Sutton R, Petersen ME. The economics of treating vasovagal syncope. *PACE* 1997; 20: 849–850.

Nyman J, Krahn A, Bland P, Criffiths S, Manda V. The costs of recurrent syncope of unknown origin in elderly patients. *PACE* 1999; 22: 1386–1394.

Risk stratification

Kapoor W. Evaluation and outcome of patients with syncope. *Medicine* 1990; 69: 169–175.

Nienaber CA, Hiller S, Spielmann RP, Geiger M, Kuck KH. Syncope in hypertrophic cardiomyopathy: multivariate analysis of prognostic determinants. *J Am Coll Cardiol* 1990; 15: 948–955.

Middlekauff H, Stevenson W, Stevenson L, Saxon L. Syncope in advanced heart failure: high risk of sudden death regardless of origin of syncope. *J Am Coll Cardiol* 1993; 21: 110–116.

Kapoor WN, Hanusa B. Is syncope a risk factor for poor outcomes? Comparison of patients with and without syncope. *Am J Med* 1996; 100: 646–655.

Sheldon R, Rose S, Flanagan P, Koshman ML, Killam S. Risk factors for syncope recurrence after a positive tilt-table test in patients with syncope. *Circulation* 1996; 93: 973–981.

Martin TP, Hanusa BH, Kapoor WN. Risk stratification of patients with syncope. *Ann Emerg Med* 1997; 29(4): 459–466.

Oh JH, Hanusa BH, Kapoor WN. Do symptoms predict cardiac arrhythmias and mortality in patients with syncope? *Arch Intern Med* 1999; 159(4): 375–380.

Martin TP, Hanusa BH, Kapoor WN. Risk stratification of patients with syncope. *Ann Emerg Med* 1997; 29(4): 459–466.

Rose MS, Koshman ML, Spreng S, Sheldon R. The relationship between health related quality of life and frequency of spells in patients with syncope. *J Clin Epidemiol* 2000; 35: 1209–1216.

Benditt DG, Brignole M. Syncope: is a diagnosis a diagnosis? *J Am Coll Cardiol* 2003; 41: 791–794.

Haver KE. Discovering the cause of syncope. A guide to the focused evaluation. *Postgrad Med* 2003; 113: 31–38.

Initial evaluation

Hoefnagels WAJ, Padberg GW, Overweg J *et al.* Transient loss of consciousness: the value of the history for distinguishing seizure from syncope. *J Neurol* 1991; 238: 39–43.

Calkins H, Shyr Y, Frumin H, Schork A, Morady F. The value of clinical history in the differentiation of syncope due to ventricular tachycardia, atrioventricular block and neurocardiogenic syncope. *Am J Med* 1995; 98: 365–373.

Linzer M, Yang EH, Estes III M *et al.* Diagnosing syncope. Part 1: Value of history, physical examination, and electrocardiography. *Ann Intern Med* 1997; 126: 989–996.

Kapoor WH. Syncope. *N Engl J Med* 2000; 343: 1856–1862.

Farwell D, Sulke N. How do we diagnose syncope? *J Cardiovasc Electrophysiol* 2001; 13: S9–S13.

Alboni P, Brignole M, Menozzi C *et al.* The diagnostic value of history in patients with syncope with or without heart disease. *J Am Coll Cardiol* 2001; 37: 1921–1928.

Sheldon R, Rose S, Ritchie D *et al.* Historical criteria that distinguish syncope from seizures. *J Am Coll Cardiol.* 2002; 40: 142–148.

Donateo P, Brignole M, Alboni P *et al.* A standardised conventional evaluation of the mechanism of syncope in patients with bundle-branch block. *Europace* 2002; 4: 357–360.

Syncope evaluation unit

Kenny RA, O'Shea D, Walker HF. Impact of a dedicated syncope and falls facility for older adults on emergency beds. *Age Ageing* 2002; 31: 272–275.

Shaw FE, Bond J, Richardson DA *et al.* Multi-factorial intervention after a fall in older people with cognitive impairment and dementia presenting to the accident and emergency department. *Br Med J* 2003; 326: 73–77.

Croci F, Brignole M, Alboni P *et al.* The application of a standardised strategy of evaluation in patients referred to three syncope units. *Europace* 2002; 4: 351–356.

Brignole M, Disertori M, Menozzi C *et al.* The management of syncope referred for emergency to general hospitals with and without syncope unit facility. (in press).

Diagnostic testing

Ambulatory electrocardiography/implantable ECG recorders

Bass EB, Curtiss EJ, Arena VC *et al.* The duration of Holter monitoring in patients with syncope: is 24 hours enough? *Arch Intern Med* 1990; 150: 1073–1078.

Linzer M, Pritchett ELC, Pontinen M, McCarthy E, Divine GW. Incremental diagnostic yield of loop electrocardiographic recorders in unexplained syncope. *Am J Cardiol* 1990; 66: 214–219.

Krahn A, Klein GJ, Yee R, Norris C. Final results from a pilot study with an implantable loop recorder to determine the etiology of syncope in patients with negative non-invasive and invasive testing. *Am J Cardiol* 1998; 82: 117–119.

Krahn AD, Klein GJ, Yee R, Takle-Newhouse T, Norris C. Use of an extended monitoring strategy in patients with problematic syncope. Reveal Investigators. *Circulation* 1999; 26: 99: 406–410.

Seidl K, Ramekan M, Breuning S *et al.* Diagnostic assessment of recurrent unexplained syncope with a new subcutaneously implantable loop recorder. *Europace* 2000: 2; 256–262.

Moya A, Brignole M, Menozzi C, Garcia-Civera R, Tognarini S, Mont L, Botto G, Giada F, Cornacchia D, and ISSUE Investigators. Mechanism of syncope in patients with isolated syncope and in patients with tilt-positive syncope. *Circulation* 2001; 104: 1261–1267.

Brignole M, Menozzi C, Moya A *et al.* Mechanism of syncope in patients with bundle branch block and negative electrophysiologic test. *Circulation* 2001; 104: 2045–2050.

Krahn A, Klein GJ, Yee R, Skanes AC. Randomized assessment of syncope trial. Conventional diagnostic testing versus a prolonged monitoring strategy. *Circulation* 2001; 104: 46–51.

Menozzi C, Brignole M, Garcia-Civera R *et al.* Mechanism of syncope in patients with heart disease and negative electrophysiologic test. *Circulation* 2002; 105: 2741–2745.

Tilt-table testing—clinical application, protocols, limitations

Fitzpatrick AP, Theodorakis G, Vardas P, Sutton R. Methodology of head-up tilt testing in patients with unexplained syncope. *J Am Coll Cardiol* 1991; 17: 125–130.

Sheldon R, Killam S. Methodology of isoproterenol-tilt table testing in patients with syncope. *J Am Coll Cardiol* 1992; 19: 773–779.

Kapoor WN, Brant N. Evaluation of syncope by upright tilt testing with isoproterenol. A nonspecific test. *Ann Intern Med* 1992; 116: 358–363.

Sheldon R, Splawinski J, Killam S. Reproducibility of isoproterenol tilt-table tests in patients with syncope. *Am J Cardiol* 1992; 69: 1300–1305.

Grubb BP, Wolfe D, Tenesy Armos P, Hahn H, Elliot L. Reproducibility of head upright tilt-table test in patients with syncope. *PACE* 1992; 15: 1477–1481.

De Buitler M, Grogan EW Jr, Picone MF, Casteen JA. Immediate reproducibility of the tilt table test in adults with unexplained syncope. *Am J Cardiol* 1993; 71: 304–307.

Brooks R, Ruskin JN, Powell AC *et al.* Prospective evaluation of day-to-day reproducibility of upright tilt-table testing in unexplained syncope. *Am J Cardiol* 1993; 71: 1289–1292.

Blanc JJ, Mansourati J, Maheu B, Boughaleb D, Genet L. Reproducibility of a positive passive upright tilt test at a seven-day interval in patients with syncope. *Am J Cardiol* 1993 15; 72: 469–471.

Gaggioli G, Bottoni N, Mureddu R *et al.* Effects of chronic vasodilator therapy to enhance susceptibility to vasovagal syncope during upright tilt testing. *Am J Cardiol* 1997; 80: 1092–1094.

Kapoor WN, Smith M, Miller NL. Upright tilt testing in evaluating syncope: a comprehensive literature review. *Am J Med* 1994; 97: 78–88.

Raviele A, Gasparini G, Di Pede F *et al.* Nitroglycerin infusion during upright tilt: a new test for the diagnosis of vasovagal syncope. *Am Heart J* 1994; 127: 103–111.

McIntosh SJ, Lawson J, Kenny RA. Intravenous cannulation alters the specificity of head-up tilt testing for vasovagal syncope in elderly patients. *Age Ageing* 1994; 63: 58–65.

Moya A, Permanyer-Miralda G, Sagrista-Sauleda J *et al.* Limitations of head-up tilt test for evaluating the efficacy of therapeutic interventions in patients with vasovagal syncope: results of a controlled study of etilefrine versus placebo. *J Am Coll Cardiol* 1995; 25: 65–69.

Tonnesen G, Haft J, Fulton J, Rubenstein D. The value of tilt testing with isoproterenol in determining therapy in adults with syncope and presyncope of unexplained origin. *Arch Intern Med* 1994; 154: 1613–1617.

Kapoor WN, Fortunato M, Hanusa SH, Schulberg HC. Psychiatric illnesses in patients with syncope. *Am J Med* 1995: 99; 505–512.

Morillo CA, Klein GJ, Zandri S, Yee R. Diagnostic accuracy of a low-dose isoproterenol head-up tilt protocol. *Am Heart J* 1995; 129(5): 901–906.

Natale A, Aktar M, Jazayeri M *et al.* Provocation of hypotension during head-up tilt testing in subjects with no history of syncope or presyncope. *Circulation* 1995; 92: 54–58.

Raviele SA, Menozzi C, Brignole M *et al.* Value of head-up tilt testing potentiated with sublingual nitriglycerin to assess the origin of unexplained syncope. *Am J Cardiol* 1995; 76: 267–272.

Fitzpatrick AP, Lee RJ, Epstein LM, Lesh MD, Eisenberg S, Sheinman MM. Effect of patient characteristics on the yield of prolonged baseline head-up tilt testing and the additional yield of drug provocation. *Heart* 1996; 76: 406–411.

Ammirati F, Colivicchi F, Biffi A, Magris B, Pandozi C, Santini M. Head-up tilt testing potentiated with low-dose sublingual isosorbide dinitrate: A simplified time-saving approach for the evaluation of unexplained syncope. *Am Heart J* 1998; 135: 671–676.

Voice RA, Lurie KG, Sakaguchi S, Rector TS, Benditt DG. Comparison of tilt angles and provocative agents (edrophonium and isoproterenol) to improve head-upright tilt-table testing. *Am J Cardiol* 1998; 81: 346–351.

Del Rosso A, Bartoli P, Bartoletti A *et al.* Shortened head-up tilt testing potentiated with sublingual nitroglycerin in patients with unexplained syncope *Am Heart J* 1998; 135: 564–570.

Natale A, Sra J, Akhtar M *et al.* Use of sublingual nitroglycerin in patients with unexplained syncope. *Am Heart J* 1998; 135: 564–570.

Imholz BPM, Wieling W, van Montfrans GA, Wesseling KH. Fifteen years experience with finger arterial pressure monitoring: assessment of the technology. *Cardiovasc Res* 1998; 38: 605–616.

Bartoletti A, Gaggioli G, Bottoni N *et al.* Head-up tilt testing potentiated with oral nitroglycerin. A randomized trial of the contribution of a drug-free phase and a nitroglycerin phase in the diagnosis of neurally mediated syncope. *Europace* 1999; 1: 183–186.

Foglia Manzillo G, Giada F, Beretta S, Corrado G, Santarone M, Raviele A. Reproducibility of head-up tilt testing potentiated with sublingual nitroglycerin in patients with unexplained syncope. *Am J Cardiol* 1999; 84: 284–288.

Raviele A, Giada F, Brignole M *et al.* Diagnostic accuracy of sublingual nitroglycerin test and low-dose isoproterenol test in patients with unexplained syncope. A comparative study. *Am J Cardiol* 2000; 85: 1194–1198.

Theodorakis G, Markianos M, Zarvalis E *et al.* Provocation of neurocardiogenic syncope by clomipramine administration during the head-up tilt test in vasovagal syncope. *J Am Coll Cardiol* 2000; 36: 174–178.

Foglia-Manzillo G, Romano M, Corrado G *et al.* Reproducibility of asystole during head-up tilt testing in patients with neurally mediated syncope. *Europace* 2002; 4: 365–368.

Electrophysiologic testing
Lacroix D, Dubuc M, Kus T, Savard P, Shenasa M, Nadeau R. Evaluation of arrhythmic causes of syncope: correlation between Holter monitoring, electrophysiologic testing, and body surface potential mapping. *Am Heart J* 1991; 122: 1346–1352.

Sra J, Anderson A, Sheikh S *et al.* Unexplained syncope evaluated by electrophysiologic studies and head-up tilt testing. *Ann Intern Med* 1991; 114: 1013–1019.

Moazez F, Peter T, Simonson J, Mandel W, Vaughn C, Gang E. Syncope of unknown origin: clinical, noninvasive, and electrophysiologic determinants of arrhythmia induction and symptom recurrence during long-term follow-up. *Am Heart J* 1991; 121: 81–88.

Gaggioli G, Bottoni N, Brignole M *et al.* Progression to second or third-degree atrioventricular block in patients electrostimulated for bundle branch block: a long-term study. *G Ital Cardiol* 1994: 24: 409–416.

Bergfeldt L, Edvardsson N, Rosenqvist M, Vallin H, Edhag O. Atrioventricular block progression in patients with bifascicular block assessed by repeated electrocardiography and a bradycardia-detecting pacemaker. *Am J Cardiol* 1994; 74: 1129–1132.

Englund A, Bergfeldt L, Rehnqvist N, Åström H, Rosenqvist M. Diagnostic value of programmed ventricular stimulation in patients with bifascicular block: a prospective study of patients with and without syncope. *J Am Coll Cardiol* 1995; 26: 1508–1515.

Brignole M, Menozzi C, Bottoni N *et al.* Mechanisms of syncope caused by transient bradycardia and the diagnostic value of electrophysiologic testing and cardiovascular reflexivity maneuvers. *Am J Cardiol* 1995; 76: 273–278.

Petrac D, Radic B, Birtic K, Gjurovic J. Prospective evaluation of infrahisal second-degree AV block induced by atrial pacing in the presence of chronic bundle branch block and syncope. *PACE Pacing Clin Electrophysiol* 1996,19: 679–687.

Bergfeldt L, Vallin H, Rosenqvist M, Insulander P, Åström H, Nordlander R. Sinus node recovery time assessment revisited: role of pharmacological blockade of the autonomic nervous system. *J Cardiovasc Electrophysiol* 1996; 7: 95–101.

Englund A, Bergfeldt L, Rosenqvist M. Pharmacological stress testing of the His-Purkinje system in patients with bifascicular block. *PACE* 1998; 21: 1979–1987.

Menozzi C, Brignole M, Alboni P *et al.* The natural course of untreated sick sinus syndrome and identification of the variables predictive of unfavourable outcome. *Am J Cardiol* 1998; 82: 1205–1209.

Link M, Kim KM, Homoud M, Estes III M, Wang P. Long-term outcome of patients with syncope associated with coronary artery disease and a non diagnostic electrophysiological evaluation. *Am J Cardiol* 1999; 83: 1334–1337.

Olshansky B, Hahn EA, Hartz VL, Prater SP, Mason JW. Clinical significance of syncope in the electrophysiologic study versus electrocardiographic monitoring (ESVEM) trial. *Am Heart J* 1999; 137: 878–886.

Brignole M, Menozzi C, Moya A *et al.* The mechanism of syncope in patients with bundle branch block and negative electrophysiologic test. *Circulation* 2001, 104: 2045–2050.

Menozzi C, Brignole M, Garcia-Civera R *et al.* Mechanism of syncope in patients with heart disease and negative electrophysiologic test. *Circulation* 2002; 105; 2741–2745.

ATP/adenosine test

Shen WK, Hammil S, Munger T *et al.* Adenosine: potential modulator for vasovagal syncope. *J Am Coll Cardiol* 1996; 28: 146–154.

Flammang D, Church T, Waynberger M, Chassing A, Antiel M. Can adenosine 5′ triphosphate be used to select treatment in severe vasovagal syndrome ? *Circulation* 1997; 96: 1201–1208.

Brignole M, Gaggioli G, Menozzi C *et al.* Adenosine-induced atrioventricular block in patients with unexplained syncope. The diagnostic value of ATP test. *Circulation* 1997; 96: 3921–3927.

Flammang D, Chassing A, Donal E, Hamani D, Erickson M, Mc Carville S. Reproducibility of the 5′ triphosphate test in vasovagal syndrome. *J Cardiovasc Electrophysiol* 1998; 9: 1161–1166.

Flammang D, Erickson M, Mc Carville S, Church T, Hamani D, Donal E. Contribution of head-up tilt testing and ATP testing in assessing the mechanisms of vaso vagal syndrome. Preliminary results and potential therapeutic implications. *Circulation* 1999; 99: 2427–2433.

Mittal S, Stein K, Markowitz S *et al.* Induction of neurally mediated syncope with adenosine. *Circulation* 1999; 99: 1318–1324.

Brignole M, Gaggioli G, Menozzi C *et al.* Clinical features of adenosine sensitive syncope and tilt-induced vasovagal syncope. *Heart* 2000; 83: 24–28.

Signal-averaged ECG and related recordings

Steinberg JS, Prystowsky E, Freedman RA *et al.* Use of the signal-averaged electrocardiogram for predicting inducible ventricular tachycardia in patients with unexplained syncope: relation to clinical variables in a multivariate analysis. *J Am Coll Cardiol* 1994; 23: 99–106.

Echocardiography

Alam M, Silverman N. Apical left ventricular lipoma presenting as syncope. *Am Heart J* 1993; 125: 1788–1790.

Recchia D, Barzilai B. Echocardiography in the evaluation of patients with syncope. *J Gen Intern Med* 1995; 10: 649–655.

Panther R, Mahmood S, Gal R. Echocardiography in the diagnostic evaluation of syncope. *J Am Soc Echocardiogr* 1998; 11: 294–298.

Clinical trial techniques

Ammirati F, Colivicchi F, Santini M. Diagnosing syncope in clinical practice: implementation of a simplified diagnostic algorithm in a multicentre prospective trial. *Eur Heart J* 2000; 21: 935–940.

Sheldon R, Rose R. Components of clinical trials for vasovagal syncope. *Europace* 2001; 3: 233–240.

Specific conditions

Neurally mediated reflex syncope

Vasovagal syncope

Sutton R, Petersen M, Brignole M, Raviele A, Menozzi C, Giani P. Proposed classification for tilt induced vasovagal syncope. *Eur J Cardiac Pacing Electrophysiol* 1992; 3: 180–183.

Kapoor WN. Evaluation and management of the patient with syncope. *JAMA* 1992; 268: 2553–2560.

Menozzi C, Brignole M, Lolli G *et al.* Follow-up of asystolic episodes in patients with cardioinhibitory, neurally mediated syncope and VVI pacemaker. *Am J Cardiol* 1993; 72: 1152–1155.

Leitch J, Klein G, Yee R, Murdick C, Teo WS. Neurally mediated syncope and atrial fibrillation. *N Engl J Med* 1991; 324: 495–496.

Raviele A, Brignole M, Sutton R *et al.* Effect of etilefrine in preventing syncopal recurrence in patients with vasovagal syncope: a double-blind, randomized, placebo-controlled trial. The Vasovagal Syncope International Study. *Circulation* 1999; 99(11): 1452–1457.

Sutton R, Brignole M, Menozzi C *et al.* Dual-chamber pacing in treatment of neurally mediated tilt-positive cardioinhibitory syncope. Pacemaker versus no therapy: a multicentre randomized study. *Circulation* 2000; 102: 294–299.

Brignole M, Menozzi C, Del Rosso A *et al.* New classification of haemodynamics of vaso-vagal syncope: beyond the VASIS classification. Analysis of the pre-syncopal phase of the tilt test without and with nitroglycerin challenge. *Europace* 2000; 2: 66–76.

Alboni P, Dinelli M, Gruppillo P *et al.* Haemodynamic changes early in prodromal symptoms of vasovagal syncope. *Europace* 2002; 4: 311–316.

Carotid sinus syndrome

Brignole M, Menozzi C, Lolli G, Oddone D, Gianfranchi L, Bertulla A. Validation of a method for choice of pacing mode in carotid sinus syndrome with or without sinus bradycardia. *PACE* 1991; 14: 196–203.

Brignole M, Menozzi C, Gianfranchi L, Oddone D, Lolli G, Bertulla A. Carotid sinus massage, eyeball compression and head-up tilt test in patients with syncope of uncertain origin and in healthy control subjects. *Am Heart J* 1991; 122: 1644–1651.

Brignole M, Menozzi C, Gianfranchi L, Oddone D, Lolli G, Bertulla A. Neurally mediated syncope detected by carotid sinus massage and head-up tilt test in sick sinus syndrome. *Am J Cardiol* 1991; 68: 1032–1036.

Brignole M, Menozzi C, Lolli G, Bottoni N, Gaggioli G. Long-term outcome of paced and non paced patients with severe carotid sinus syndrome. *Am J Cardiol* 1992; 69: 1039–1043.

Brignole M, Menozzi C. Carotid sinus syndrome: diagnosis, natural history and treatment. *Eur J Cardiac Pacing Electrophysiol* 1992; 4: 247–254.

Munro N, Mc Intosh S, Lawson J *et al.* The incidence of complications after carotid sinus massage in older patients with syncope. *J Am Geriatr Soc* 1994; 42: 1248–1251.

Gaggioli G, Brignole M, Menozzi C *et al.* Reappraisal of the vasodepressor reflex in carotid sinus syndrome. *Am J Cardiol* 1995; 75: 518–521.

Davies AG, Kenny RA. Neurological complications following carotid sinus massage. *Am J Cardiol* 1998; 81: 1256–1257.

Parry SW, Richardson D, O'Shea D, Sen B, Kenny RA. Diagnosis of carotid sinus hypersensitivity in older adults: carotid sinus massage in the upright position is essential. *Heart* 2000; 83: 22–23.

Kenny RA, Richardson DA, Steen N *et al.* Carotid sinus syndrome: a modifiable risk factor for non-accidental falls in older adults (SAFE PACE). *J Am Coll Cardiol* 2001 Nov 1; 38(5): 1491–1496.

Richardson DA, Bexton R, Shaw FE *et al.* How reproducible is the cardioinhibitory response to carotid sinus massage in fallers. *Europace* 2002; 4: 361–364.

Miscellaneous

Johnston RT, Redding V. Glossopharyngeal neuralgia associated with cardiac syncope: long term treatment with permanent pacing and carbamazepine. *Br Heart J* 1990; 36: 58–63.

Ferrante I, Artico M, Nadacci B *et al.* Glossopharyngeal neuralgia with cardiac syncope. *Neurosurgery* 1995; 36: 58–63.

Scherrer U, Vissing S, Morgan BJ, Hanson P, Victor RG. Vasovagal syncope after infusion of a vasodilator in a heart-transplant recipient. *N Engl J Med* 1990; 322: 602–604.

Fitzpatrick AP, Banner N, Cheng A, Yacoub M, Sutton R. Vasovagal syncope may occur after orthotopic heart transplantation. *J Am Coll Cardiol* 1993; 21: 1132–1137.

Morgan-Hughes NJ, Kenny RA, Scott CD, Dark JH, McComb JM. Vasodepressor reactions after orthotopic cardiac transplantation: relationship to reinnervation status. *Clin Autonom Res* 1994; 4: 125–129.

Secher NH, Sander-Jensen K, Werner C, Warberg J, Bie P. Bradycardia, a severe but reversible hypovolemic shock in man. *Circ Shock* 1984; 14: 267–274.

Secher NH, Jensen KS, Werner J, Warberg J, Schwartz TW. Vagal slowing of the heart during hemorrhage: observations from 20 consecutive hypotensive patients. *Brit Med J* 1986; 292: 365–366.

Sakaguchi S, Shultz JJ, Remole SC *et al.* Syncope associated with exercise, a manifestation of neurally mediated syncope. *Am J Cardiol* 1995; 75: 476–481.

Calkins H, Seifert M, Morady F. Clinical presentation and long-term follow-up of athletes with exercise-induced vasodepressor syncope. *Am Heart J* 1995; 129: 1159–1164.

Orthostatic syncope

Smit AAJ, Halliwill JR, Low PA, Wieling W. Topical Review. Pathophysiological basis of orthostatic hypotension in autonomic failure. *J Physiol* 1999; 519: 1–10.

Omboni S, Smit AA, van Lieshout JJ, Settels JJ, Langewouters GJ, Wieling W. Mechanisms underlying the impairment in orthostatic intolerance after nocturnal recumbency in patients with autonomic failure. *Clin Sci* 2001; 101: 609–618.

Wieling W, Harms MPM, Kortz RAM, Linzer M. Initial orthostatic hypotension as a cause of recurrent syncope: a case report. *Clin Autonom Res* 2001; 11: 269–270.

Grubb BP, Kanjwal Y, Kosinski DJ. The postural orthostatic tachycardia syndrome; Current concepts in pathophysiology, diagnosis and management. *J Intervent Cardiac Electrophysiol* 2001; 5: 9–16.

Jordan J. Acute effects of water on blood pressure—what do we know. *Clin Autonom Res* 2002; 12: 250–255.

Mukai S, Lipsitz LA. Orthostatic hypotension. *Clin Geriatr Med* 2002; 18: 253–268.

Schatz IJ. Orthostatic hypotension predicts mortality. Lessons from the Honolulu heart program. *Clin Autonom Res* 2002; 12; 223–224.

Cardiac arrhythmias as primary cause

See also "Electrophysiologic testing".

Long QT syndromes/Brugada syndrome

Schwartz PJ *et al.* Stress and sudden death: the case of the long QT syndrome. *Circulation* 1991; 83(Supp II): 71–80.

Brugada J, Brugada P. Further characterization of the syndrome of right bundle branch block, ST segment elevation and sudden cardiac death. *J Cardiovasc Electrophysiol* 1997; 8: 325–331.

Alings M, Wilde A. "Brugada" syndrome. Clinical data and suggested pathophysiological mechanism. *Circulation* 1999; 99: 666–673.

Brugada J, Brugada P, Brugada R. The syndrome of right bundle branch block ST segment elevation in V1 to V3 and sudden death: the Brugada syndrome. *Europace* 1999; 1: 156–166.

Barbey JT, Lazzara R, Zipes DP. Spontaneous adverse event reports of serious ventricular arrhythmias, QT prolongation, syncope, and sudden death in patients treated with cisapride. *J Cardiovasc Pharmacol Therap* 2002; 7: 65–76.

Syncope with myocardial ischemia

Havranek EP, Dunbar DN. Exertional syncope caused by left main coronary artery spasm. *Am Heart J* 1992; 123: 792–794.

Watanabe K, Inomata T, Miyakita Y *et al.* Electrophysiologic study and ergonovine provocation of coronary spasm in unexplained syncope. *Jpn Heart J* 1993; 34: 171–182.

Kovac JD, Murgatroyd FD, Skehan JD. Recurrent syncope due to complete atrioventricular block, a rare presenting symptom of otherwise silent coronary artery disease: successful treatment by PTCA. *Cathet Cardiovasc Diagn* 1997; 42: 216–218.

Ascheim DD, Markowitz SM, Lai H, Engelstein ED, Stein KM, Lerman BB. Vasodepressor syncope due to subclinical myocardial ischemia. *J Cardiovasc Electrophysiol* 1997; 8: 215–221.

Syncope with exercise (neural reflex, primary cardiac arrhythmias)

Greci ED, Ramsdale DR. Exertional syncope in aortic stenosis: evidence to support inappropriate left ventricular baroreceptor response. *Am Heart J* 1991; 121: 603–606.

Pavlovic S, Kocovic D, Djordjevic M *et al.* The etiology of syncope in pacemaker patients. *PACE* 1991; 14: 2086–2091.

Leitch JW, Klein GJ, Yee R *et al.* Syncope associated with supraventricular tachycardia: An expression of tachycardia or vasomotor response. *Circulation* 1992; 85: 1064–1071.

Arad M, Solomon A, Roth A, Atsmon J, Rabinowitz B. Postexercise syncope: evidence for increased activity of the sympathetic nervous system. *Cardiology* 1993; 83: 121–123.

Osswald S, Brooks R, O'Nunain SS *et al.* Asystole after exercise in healthy persons. *Ann Intern Med* 1994; 120: 1008–1011.

Sneddon JF, Scalia G, Ward DE, McKenna WJ, Camm AJ, Frenneaux MP. Exercise induced vasodepressor syncope. *Br Heart J* 1994; 71: 554–557.

Byrne JM, Marais HJ, Cheek GA. Exercise-induced complete heart block in a patient with chronic bifascicular block. *J Electrocardiol* 1994; 27: 339–342.

Sakaguchi S, Shultz JJ, Remole SC, Adler SW, Lurie KG, Benditt DG. Syncope associated with exercise, a manifestation of neurally mediated syncope. *Am J Cardiol* 1995; 75: 476–481.

Calkins H, Seifert M, Morady F. Clinical presentation and long-term follow-up of athletes with exercise-induced vasodepressor syncope. *Am Heart J* 1995; 129: 1159–1164.

Smith GPD, Mathias CJ. Postural hypotension enhanced by exercise in patients with chronic autonomic failure. *Q J Med* 1995; 88: 251–256.

Thomson HL, Atherton JJ, Khafagi FA, Frenneaux MP. Failure to reflex venoconstriction during exercise in patients with vasovagal syncope. *Circulation* 1996; 93: 953–959.

Kosinski D, Grubb BP, Kip K, Hahn H. Exercise-induced neurocardiogenic syncope. *Am Heart J* 1996; 132: 451–452.

Neurologic disorders

Davis TL, Freemon FR. Electroencephalography should not be routine in the evaluation of syncope in adults. *Arch Intern Med* 1990; 1 50: 2027–2029.

Van Donselaar CA, Geerts AT, Schimsheimer RJ. Usefullness of an aura for classification of a first generalised seizure. *Epilepsia* 1990; 31: 529–535.

Hoefnagels WA, Padberg GW, Overweg J, Roos RA, van Dijk JG, Karnphuisen HA. Syncope or seizure? The diagnostic value of the EEG and hyperventilation test in transient loss of consciousness. *J Neurol Neurosurg Psychiatr* 1991; 54: 953–956.

Davidson E, Rotenbeg Z, Fuchs J, Weinberger I, Agmon J. Transient ischemic attack-related syncope. *Clin Cardiol* 1991; 14: 141–144.

Guilleminault C, Gelb M. Clinical aspects and features of cataplexy. In: Fahn S, Hallett M, Luders HO, Marsden CD, eds. *Negative Motor Phenomena* 1995; Vol. 67: 65–77.

Gosselin C, Walker PM. Subclavian steal syndrome. Existence, clinical features, diagnosis, management. *Semin Vasc Surg* 1996; 9: 93–97.

Wenning GK, Tison F, Shlomo YB, Daniel SE, Quinn NP. Multiple system atrophy: a review of 203 pathologically proven cases. *Mov Dis* 1997; 12: 133–147.

Bannister R, Mathias C. Introduction and classification of autonomic disorders. In: Mathias CJ, Bannister R, eds. *Autonomic Failure*, 4th edn. Oxford University Press, Oxford, 1999: xvii–xxii.

Tonkin AL, Frewin DB. Drugs, toxins and chemicals that alter autonomic function. In: Mathias CJ, Bannister R, eds. *Autonomic Failure*, 4th edn. Oxford University Press, Oxford, 1999: 527–533.

Mathias CJ, Polinsky RJ. Separating the primary autonomic failure syndromes, multiple system atrophy, and pure autonomic failure from Parkinson's disease. In: Stern GM, ed. *Parkinson's Disease: Advances in Neurology*, Vol 80. Lippincott Philadelphia 1999.

Syncope in childhood and adolescents

Paul T, Guccione P, Garson A Jr. Relation of syncope in young patients with Wolff–Parkinson–White syndrome to rapid ventricular response during atrial fibrillation. *Am J Cardiol* 1990; 65: 318–321.

Camfield PR, Camfield CS. Syncope in childhood: a case control clinical study of the familial tendency to faint. *Can J Neurol Sci* 1990; 17(3): 306–308.

Chandar JS, Wolff GS, Garson A Jr *et al.* Ventricular arrhythmias in postoperative tetralogy of Fallot. *Am J Cardiol* 1990; 65: 655–661.

Perry JC, Garson A Jr. The child with recurrent syncope: autonomic function testing and beta-adrenergic hypersensitivity. *J Am Coll Cardiol* 1991; 17: 1168–1171.

Dambrink JHA, Imholz BPM, Karemaker JM, Wieling W. Circulatory adaptation to orthostatic stress in healthy 10–14 year old children investigated in a general practice. *Clin Sci* 1991; 81: 51–58.

Dambrink JHA, Imholz BPM, Karemaker JM, Wieling W. Postural and transient hypotension in two healthy teenagers. *Clin Autonom Res* 1991; 1: 281–287.

Grubb BP, Temesy-Armos P, Moore J, Wolfe D, Hahn H, Elliott L. The use of head-upright tilt table testing in the evaluation and management of syncope in children and adolescents. *Pacing Clin Electrophysiol* 1992; 15: 742–748.

Konig D, Linzer M, Pontinen M, Divine GW. Syncope in young adults: evidence for a combined medical and psychiatric approach. *J Intern Med* 1992; 232: 169–176.

Garson A Jr, Dick M, Fournier A *et al.* The long QT syndrome in children. An international study of 287 patients. *Circulation* 1993; 87(6): 1866–1872.

Strieper MJ, Campbell RMJ. Efficacy of alpha-adrenergic agonist therapy for prevention of pediatric neurocardiogenic syncope. *Am Coll Cardiol* 1993; 22: 594–597.

O'Marcaigh AS, MacLellan-Tobert SG, Porter CJ. Tilt-table testing and oral metoprolol therapy in young patients with unexplained syncope. *Pediatrics* 1994; 93: 278–283.

Lucet V, Grau F, Denjoy I *et al.* Long term course of catecholaminergic polymorphic ventricular tachycardia in children. Apropos of 20 cases with an 8 year-follow-up. *Arch Pediatr* 1994; 1: 26–32.

Daliento L, Turrini P, Nava A *et al.* Arrhythmogenic right ventricular cardiomyopathy in young versus adult patients: similarities and differences. *J Am Coll Cardiol* 1995; 25: 655–664.

Michaelsson M, Jonzon A, Riesenfeld T. Isolated congenital complete atrioventricular block in adult life. *Circulation* 1995; 92: 442–449.

De Jong-de Vos van Steenwijk CCE, Wieling W *et al.* Incidence and hemodynamics of near-fainting in healthy 6–16 year old subjects. *J Am Coll Cardiol* 1995; 25: 1615–1621.

De Jong-de Vos van Steenwijk CCE, Wieling W, Harms MPM, Wesseling KH. Variability of near-fainting responses in healthy 6–16-year-old subjects. *Clin Sci* 1997; 93: 205–211.

Driscoll DJ, Jacobsen SJ, Porter CJ, Wollan PC. Syncope in children and adolescents. *J Am Coll Cardiol* 1997; 29: 1039–1045.

McHarg ML, Shinnar S, Rascoff H, Walsh CA. Syncope in childhood. *Pediatr Cardiol* 1997; 18: 367–371.

Lenk M, Alehan D, Ozme S, Celiker A, Ozer S. The role of serotonin re-uptake inhibitors in preventing recurrent unexplained childhood syncope—a preliminary report. *Eur J Pediatr* 1997; 156: 747–750.

Lewis DA, Zlotocha J, Henke L, Dhala A. Specificity of head-up tilt testing in adolescents: effect of various degrees of tilt challenge in normal control subjects. *J Am Coll Cardiol* 1997; 30: 1057–1060.

Deal BJ, Strieper M, Scagliotti D *et al.* The medical therapy of cardioinhibitory syncope in pediatric patients. *Pacing Clin Electrophysiol* 1997; 20: 1759–1761.

Lewis DA, Dhala A. Syncope in the pediatric patient. The cardiologist's perspective. *Pediatr Clin North Am* 1999; 46(2): 205–219.

Levine MM. Neurally mediated syncope in children: results of tilt testing, treatment, and long-term follow-up. *Pediatr Cardiol* 1999; 20: 331–335.

Saul JP. Syncope: etiology, management, and when to refer. *J S C Med Assoc* 1999; 95: 385–387.

McLeod KA, Wilson N, Hewitt J *et al.* Cardiac pacing for severe childhood neurally mediated syncope with reflex anoxic seizures. *Heart* 1999; 82: 721–725.

Tanaka H, Yamaguchi H, Matashima R, Tamai H. Instantaneous orthostatic hypotension in children and adolescents: a new entity of orthostatic intolerance. *Pediatr Res* 1999; 46: 691–697.

Syncope in older adults and the elderly

Kenny RA, Traynor G. Carotid sinus syndrome—clinical characteristics in elderly patients. *Age Ageing* 1991; 20: 449–454.

Tonkin A, Wing LMH, Morris MJ, Kapoor V. Afferent baroreflex dysfunction and age-related orthostatic hypotension. *Clin Sci* 1991; 81: 531–538.

Wieling W, Veerman DP, Dambrink JHA, Imholz BPM. Disparities in circulatory adjustment to standing between young and elderly subjects explained by pulse contour analysis. *Clin Sci* 1992; 83: 149–155.

Brignole M, Oddone D, Cogorno S *et al.* Long term outcome in symptomatic carotid sinus hypersensitivity. *Am Heart J*, 1992; 123: 687–692.

McIntosh SJ, da Costa D, Kenny RA. Outcome of an integrated approach to the investigation of dizziness, falls and syncope in elderly patients referred to a syncope clinic. *Age Ageing* 1993; 22: 53–58.

McIntosh SJ, Lawson J, Kenny RA. Clinical characteristics of vasodepressor, cardioinhibitory and mixed carotid sinus syndrome in the elderly. *Am J Med* 1993; 95: 203–208.

Tinetti ME, Mendes de Leon CF, Doncette JT, Baker DI. Fear of falling and fall related efficacy. *J Gerontol* 1994; 49: 140–147.

Tonkin A, Wing L. Effects of age and isolated systolic hypertension on cardiovascular reflexes. *Hypertension* 1994; 12: 1083–1088.

Cumming SR, Nevitt MC, Browner WS *et al*. The study of osteoporotic fractures research group. *N Engl J Med* 1995; 332: 767–773.

Ward C, Kenny RA. Reproducibility of orthostatic hypotension in symptomatic elderly. *Am J Med* 1996; 100: 418–411.

Hussain RM, McIntosh SJ, Lawson J, Kenny RA. Fludrocortisone in the treatment of hypotensive disorders in the elderly. *Heart* 1996; 76: 507–509.

Shaw FE, Kenny RA. Overlap between syncope and falls in the elderly. *Postgrad Med J* 1997; 73: 635–639.

Shaw FE, Kenny RA. Can falls in patients with dementia be prevented. *Age Ageing* 1997; 27: 1–7.

Masaki KH, Schatz IJ, Burchfiel CM *et al*. Orthostatic hypotension predicts mortality in elderly men: the Honolulu heart program. *Circulation* 1998; 98: 2290–2295.

Ward C, McIntosh SJ, Kenny RA. Carotid sinus hypersensitivity—a modifiable risk factor for fractured neck of femur. *Age Ageing* 1999; 28: 127–133.

Ballard C, Shaw F, McKeith I, Kenny RA. Prevalence, assessment and associations of falls in dementia with Lewy bodies and Alzheimer's disease dementia. *Dementia* 1999; 10: 97–103.

Ballard C, Shaw F, McKeith, Kenny RA. High prevalence of neurocardiovascular instability in Alzheimer's disease and dementia with Lewy bodies; potential treatment implications. *Neurology* 1998; 51: 1760–1762.

Allcock LM, O'Shea D. Diagnostic yield and development of a neurocardiovascular investigation unit for older adults in a district hospital. *J Gerontol A Biol Med Sci* 2000; 55: M458–62.

Conditions mimicking syncope

Linzer M, Felder A, Hackel A, Perry AJ, Varia I, Melville ML. Psychiatric syncope: a new look at an old disease. *Psychosomatics* 1990; 31: 181–188.

Linzer M, Pontinen M, Gold DT, Divine GW, Felder A, Brooks WB. Impairment of physical and psychosocial function in recurrent syncope. *J Clin Epidemiol* 1991; 44: 1037–1043.

Grubb BP, Gerard G, Wolfe DA, Samoil D, Davenport CW, Homan RW. Syncope and seizure of psychogenic origin: identification with head-upright tilt table testing. *Clin Cardiol* 1992; 15: 839–842.

Kapoor W, Fortunato M, Hanusa BH, Schulberg HC. Psychiatric illnesses in patients with syncope. *Am J Med* 1995; 99: 505–551.

Kouakam C, Lacroix D, Klug D, Baux P, Marquie C, Kacet S. Prevalence and prognostic significance of psychiatric disorders in patients evaluated for recurrent unexplained syncope. *Am J Cardiol* 2002; 89: 530–535.

Personal and public safety issues

Epstein AE, Miles WM, Benditt DG, Camm AJ *et al.* Personal and public safety issues related to arrhythmias that may affect consciousness: implications for regulation and physician recommendations. *Circulation* 1996; 94: 1147–1166.

Driving and heart disease. Task Force Report. Prepared on behalf of the Task Force by MC Petch. *Eur Heart J* 1998; 19: 1165–1177.

Sutton R. Vasovagal syncope: prevalence and presentation. An algorithm of management in the aviation environment. *Eur Heart J* (Supp) 1999: D109–13.

Treatment options

Neurally mediated reflex syncope

Carotid sinus syndrome

Deschamps D, Richard A, Citron B, Chaperon A, Binon JP, Ponsonaille J. Hypersensibilité sino-carotidienne. Evolution à moyen et à long terme des patients traités par stimulation ventriculaire. *Arch Mal Coeur* 1990; 83: 63–67.

Grubb BP, Samoil D, Kosinski D, Temesy-Armos P, Akpunonu B. The use of serotonin reuptake inhibitors for the treatment of carotid sinus hypersensitivity syndrome unresponsive to dual chamber pacing. *PACE* 1994; 17: 1434–1436.

Brignole M, Menozzi C, Gaggioli G *et al.* Effects of vasodilator therapy in patients with carotid sinus hypersensitivity. *Am Heart J* 1998; 136: 264–268.

Vasovagal syncope

Physical maneuvers/fluid/volume

Ector H, Reybrouck T, Heidbuchel H, Gewillig M, Van de Werf F. Tilt training: a new treatment for recurrent neurocardiogenic syncope or severe orthostatic intolerance. *PACE* 1998; 21: 193–196.

Younoszai AK, Franklin WH, Chan DP, Cassidy SC, Allen HD. Oral fluid therapy. A promising treatment for vasodepressor syncope. *Arch Pediatr Adolescent Med* 1998; 152: 165–168.

Di Girolamo E, Di Iorio C, Leonzio L, Sabatini P, Barsotti A. Usefulness of a tilt training program for the prevention of refractory neurocardiogenic syncope in adolescents. A controlled study. *Circulation* 1999; 100: 1798–1801.

Reybrouck T, Heidbuchel H, Van De Werf F, Ector H. Long-term follow-up results of tilt training therapy in patients with recurrent neurocardiogenic syncope. *PACE* 2002; 25: 1441–1446.

Abe H, Kondo S, Kohshi K, Nakashima Y. Usefulness of orthostatic self-training for the prevention of neurocardiogenic syncope. *PACE* 2002; 25: 1454–1458.

Kerdiet CTP, van Dijk N, Linzer M, van Lieshout JJ, Wieling W. Management of vasovagal syncope: Controlling or aborting faints by leg crossing and muscle tensing. *Circulation* 2002; 106: 1684–1689.

Pharmacologic treatment

Milstein S, Buetikofer J, Dunnigan A, Benditt DG, Gornick C, Reyes WJ. Usefulness of disopyramide for prevention of upright tilt-induced hypotension-bradycardia. *Am J Cardiol* 1990; 65: 1339–1344.

Fitzpatrick AP, Ahmed R, Williams S *et al*. A randomized trial of medical therapy in malignant vasovagal syndrome or neurally mediated bradycardia/hypotension syndrome. *Eur J Cardiac Pacing Electrophysiol* 1991; 1: 191–202.

Brignole M, Menozzi C, Gianfranchi L *et al*. A controlled trial of acute and long–term medical therapy in tilt-induced neurally mediated syncope. *Am J Cardiol* 1992; 70: 339–342.

Grubb BP, Wolfe D, Samoil D, Temesy-Armos P, Hahn H, Elliott L. Usefulness of fluoxetine hydrochloride for prevention of resistant upright tilt induced syncope. *PACE* 1993; 16: 458–464.

Muller G, Deal B, Strasburger JF, Benson DW Jr. Usefulness of metoprolol for unexplained syncope and positive response to tilt testing in young persons. *Am J Cardiol* 1993; 71: 592–595.

Kelly PA, Mann DE, Adler SW, Fuenzalida CE, Reiter MJ. Low dose disopyramide often fails to prevent neurogenic syncope during head-up tilt testing. *PACE* 1994; 17: 573–576.

Mahanonda N, Bhuripanyo K, Kangkagate C *et al*. Randomized double-blind, placebo-controlled trial of oral atenolol in patients with unexplained syncope and positive upright tilt table test results. *Am Heart J* 1995; 130: 1250–1253.

Cohen MB, Snow JS, Grasso V *et al*. Efficacy of pindolol for treatment of vasovagal syncope. *Am Heart J* 1995; 130: 786–790.

Jhamb DK, Singh B, Sharda B, Kaul U, Goel P, Talwar KK, Wasir HS. Comparative study of the efficacy of metoprolol and verapamil in patients with syncope and positive head-up tilt test response. *Am Heart J* 1996; 132: 608–611.

Sheldon R, Rose S, Flanagan P, Koshman L, Killam S. Effects of beta blockers on the time to first syncope recurrence in patients after a positive isoproterenol tilt table test. *Am J Cardiol* 1996; 78: 536–539.

Biffi M, Boriani G, Sabbatani P *et al*. Malignant vasovagal syncope: a randomised trial of metoprolol and clonidine. *Heart* 1997; 77: 268–272.

Sra J, Maglio C, Biehl M, Dhala A *et al*. Efficacy of midodrine hydrochloride in neurocardiogenic syncope refractory to standard therapy. *J Cardiovasc Electrophysiol* 1997; 8: 42–46.

Iskos D, Dutton J, Scheinman MM, Lurie KG. Usefulness of pindolol in neurocardiogenic syncope. *Am J Cardiol*.1998; 82: 1121–1124.

Ward CR, Gray JC, Gilroy JJ, Kenny RA. Midodrine: a role in the management of neurocardiogenic syncope. *Heart* 1998; 79: 45–49.

Di Girolamo E, Di Iorio C, Sabatini P, Leonzio L, Barsotti A. Effects of different treatments vs no treatment on neurocardiogenic syncope. *Cardiologia* 1998; 43: 833–837.

Di Girolamo E, Di Iorio C, Sabatini O, Leonzio L, Barbone C, Barsotti A. Effects of paroxetine hydrochloride, a selective serotonin reuptake inhibitor, on refractory vasovagal syncope: a randomized, double-blind, placebo-controlled study. *J Am Coll Cardiol* 1999; 33: 1227–1230.

Raviele A, Brignole M, Sutton R *et al*. Effect of etilefrine in preventing syncopal recurrence in patients with vasovagal syncope: a double-blind, randomized, placebo-controlled trial. The Vasovagal Syncope International Study. *Circulation* 1999; 99(11): 1452–1457.

Madrid A, Ortega I, Rebollo GJ *et al.* Lack of efficacy of atenolol for the prevention of neurally mediated syncope in highly symptomatic population: a prospective double-blind, randomized and placebo-controlled study. *J Am Coll Cardiol* 2001; 37: 554–557.

Perez-Lugones A, Schweikert R, Pavia S, Sra J, Akhtar M, Jaeger F *et al.* Usefulness of midodrine in patients with severely symptomatic neurocardiogenic syncope: a randomized control study. *J Cardiovasc Electrophysiol* 2001; 935–938.

Pacemaker treatment

Fitzpatrick A, Theodorakis G, Ahmed R, Williams T, Sutton R. Dual chamber pacing aborts vasovagal syncope induced by head-up 60 degree tilt. *PACE* 1991; 14: 13–19.

Samoil D, Grubb BP, Brewster P, Moore J, Temesy-Armos P. Comparison of single and dual chamber pacing techniques in prevention of upright tilt induced vasovagal syncope. *Eur J Cardiac Pacing Electrophysiol* 1993; 1: 36–41.

Sra J, Jazayeri MR, Avitall B, Dhala A, Deshpande S, Blanck Z, Akhtar M. Comparison of cardiac pacing with drug therapy in the treatment of neurocardiogenic (vasovagal) syncope with bradycardia or asystole. *N Engl J Med* 1993; 328; 1085–1090.

Petersen MEV, Chamberlain-Webber R, Fizpatrick AP, Ingram A, Williams T, Sutton R. Permanent pacing for cardio-inhibitory malignant vasovagal syndrome. *Br Heart J* 1994; 71: 274–281.

El-Bedawi KM, Wahbha MAE, Hainsworth R. Cardiac pacing does not improve orthostatic tolerance in patients with vasovagal syncope. *Clin Autonom Res* 1995: 88: 463–470.

Benditt DG, Petersen M, Lurie KG, Grubb BL, Sutton R. Cardiac pacing for prevention of recurrent vasovagal syncope. *Ann Intern Med* 1995; 122: 204–209.

Benditt DG, Sutton R, Gammage M *et al.* Rate-Drop Response Investigators Group. Rate-drop response cardiac pacing for vasovagal syncope. *J Intervent Cardiac Electrophys* 1999; 3: 27–33.

Connolly SJ, Sheldon R, Roberts RS, Gent M, Vasovagal pacemaker study investigators. The North American vasovagal pacemaker study (VPS): a randomized trial of permanent cardiac pacing for the prevention of vasovagal syncope. *J Am Coll Cardiol* 1999; 33: 16–20.

Benditt DG. Cardiac pacing for prevention of vasovagal syncope (editorial). *J Am Coll Cardiol* 1999; 33: 21–23.

Sutton R, Brignole M, Menozzi C *et al.* Dual-chamber pacing in treatment of neurally mediated tilt-positive cardioinhibitory syncope. Pacemaker versus no therapy: a multicentre randomized study. *Circulation* 2000; 102: 294–299.

Ammirati F, Colivicchi F, Santini M *et al.* Permanent cardiac pacing versus medical treatment for the prevention of recurrent vasovagal syncope. A multicenter, randomized, controlled trial. *Circulation* 2001; 104: 52–56.

Raviele A, Giada F, Sutton R *et al.* The vasovagal syncope and pacing (Synpace) trial: rationale and study design. *Europace* 2001; 3: 336–341.

Miscellaneous treatment options

Khurana R, Lynch J, Craig F. A novel psychological treatment for vasovagal syncope. *Clin Autonom Res* 1997; 7: 191–197.

Van Dijk N, Velzeboer S, Destree-Vonk A, Linzer M, Wieling W. Psychological treatment of malignant vasovagal syncope due to bloodphobia. *PACE* 2001; 24: 122–124.

Orthostatic syncope

Ten Harkel ADJ, van Lieshout JJ, Wieling W. Treatment of orthostatic hypotension with sleeping in the head-up position, alone and in combination with fludrocortisone. *J Intern Med* 1992; 232: 139–145.

Van Lieshout JJ, Ten Harkel ADJ, Wieling W. Combating orthostatic dizziness in autonomic failure by physical maneuvers. *Lancet* 1992; 339: 897–898.

Wieling W, Van Lieshout JJ, Van Leeuwen AM. Physical maneuvers that reduce postural hypotension in autonomic failure. *Clin Autonom Res* 1993; 3: 57–65.

Jankovic J, Gilden JL, Hiner BC, Brown DC, Rubin M. Neurogenic orthostatic hypotension: A double-blind placebo-controlled study with midodrine. *Am J Med* 1993; 95: 38–48.

Gilden JL. Midodrine in neurogenic orthostatic hypotension. *Int Angiol* 1993; 12: 125–131.

El-Sayed H, Hainsworth R. Salt supplement increases plasma volume and orthostatic tolerance in patients with unexplained syncope. *Heart* 1996; 75: 114–115.

Kardos A, Avramov K, Dongo A, Gingl Z, Kardos L, Rudas L. Management of severe orthostatic hypotension by head-up tilt posture and administration of fludrocortisone. *Orvosi Hetilap* 1996; 43: 2407–2411.

Tanaka H, Yamaguchi H, Tamai H. Treatment of orthostatic intolerance with inflatable abdominal band. *Lancet* 1997; 349: 175.

Smit AAJ, Hardjowijono MA, Wieling W. Are portable folding chairs useful to combat orthostatic hypotension? *Ann Neurol* 1997; 42: 975–978.

Low PA, Gilden JL, Freeman R, Sheng K-N, McElligott MA. Efficacy of midrodrine vs placebo in neurogenic orthostatic hypotension. *JAMA* 1997; 13: 1046–1051.

Mtinangi BL, Hainsworth R. Early effects of oral salt on plama volume, orthostatic tolerance, and baroreceptor sensitivity in patients with syncope. *Clin Autonom Res* 1998; 8: 231–235.

Mtinangi, B. Hainsworth R. Increased orthostatic tolerance following moderate exercise training in patients with unexplained syncope. *Heart* 1998; 80: 596–600.

Mathias CJ, Kimber JR. Treatment of postural hypotension. *J Neurol Neurosurg Psychiat* 1998; 65: 285–289.

Van Lieshout JJ, Ten Harkel ADJ, Wieling W. Physiological basis of treatment of orthostatic hypotension by sleeping head-up tilt and fludrocortisone medication. *Clin Autonom Res* 2000; 10: 35–42.

Wieling W, van Lieshout JJ, Hainsworth R. Extracellular fluid volume expansion in patients with posturally related syncope. *Clin Autonom Res* 2002; 12: 243–249.

Cardiac arrhythmias as primary cause

Cardiac pacemakers

Sgarbossa EB, Pinski SL, Jaeger FJ, Trohman RG, Maloney JD. Incidence and predictors of syncope in paced patients with sick sinus syndrome. *PACE* 1992; 15: 2055–2060.

Andersen HR, Thuesen L, Bagger JP *et al.* Prospective randomised trial of atrial versus ventricular pacing in sick-sinus syndrome. *Lancet* 1994; 344: 1523–1528.

Andersen HR, Nielsen JC, Thomsen PE *et al.* Long-term follow-up of patients from a randomised trial of atrial versus ventricular pacing for sick-sinus syndrome. *Lancet* 1997; 350: 1210–1216.

Alboni P, Menozzi C, Brignole M *et al.* Effects of permanent pacemaker and oral theo-phylline in sick sinus syndrome. The THEOPACE study: a randomized controlled trial. *Circulation* 1997; 96: 260–266.

Lamas G, Orav EJ, Stambler B *et al.* Quality of life and clinical outcome in elderly patients treated with ventricular pacing as compared with dual-chamber pacing. *N Engl J Med* 1998; 338: 1097–1104.

Implantable defibrillators

Link MS, Costeas XF, Griffith JL *et al.* High incidence of appropriate implantable cardioverter-defibrillator therapy in patients with syncope of unknown etiology and inducible ventricular tachycardia. *J Am Coll Cardiol* 1997; 29: 370–375.

Militianu A, Salacata A, Seibert K *et al.* Implantable cardioverter defibrillator utilization among device recipients presenting exclusively with syncope or near-syncope. *J Cardiovasc Electrophysiol* 1997; 8: 1087–1097.

Knight B, Goyal R, Pelosi F *et al.* Outcome of patients with nonischemic dilated car-diomyopathy and unexplained syncope treated with an implantable defibrillator. *J Am Coll Cardiol* 1999; 33: 1964–1970.

Mittal S, Iwai S, Stein K *et al.* Long-term outcome of patients with unexplained syncope treated with an electrophysiologic-guided approach in the implantable cardioverter-defibrillator era. *J Am Coll Cardiol* 1999; 34: 1082–1089.

Andrews N, Fogel R, Pelargonio G, Evans J, Prystowsky E. Implantable defibrillator event rates in patients with unexplained syncope and inducible sustained ventricular tachyarrhythmias. *J Am Coll Cardiol* 1999; 34: 2023–2030.

Pires L, May L, Ravi S *et al.* Comparison of event rates and survival in patients with unexplained syncope without documented ventricular tachyarrhythmias versus patients with documented sustained ventricular tachyarrhythmias both treated with implantable cardioverter-defibrillator. *Am J Cardiol* 2000; 85: 725–728.

Fonarow G, Feliciano Z, Boyle N *et al.* Improved survival in patients with nonischemic advanced heart failure and syncope treated with an implantable cardioverter-defibrillator. *Am J Cardiol* 2000; 85: 981–985.

Index

Page numbers in *italics* represent figures, those in **bold** represent tables.